PREGNANCY
The Psychological Experience

PREGNANCY
The Psychological Experience

LIBBY LEE COLMAN, Ph.D.

ARTHUR D. COLMAN, M.D.

Revised and expanded

THE NOONDAY PRESS
Farrar, Straus and Giroux
NEW YORK

Library of Congress Cataloging-in-Publication Data
Colman, Libby Lee.
Pregnancy : the psychological experience / Libby Lee Colman and
Arthur D. Colman. — Rev. and expanded ed.
p.   cm.
Arthur D. Colman's name appears first on the earlier edition.
Includes bibliographical references (p.   ) and index.
1. Pregnancy—Psychological aspects. 2. Childbirth—Psychological
aspects. I. Colman, Arthur D., 1937–   . II. Title.
RG560.C65   1990   618.2'0019—dc20   90-7468 CIP

To Shoshana, Jonah, and Ariel

Acknowledgments

THE AUTHORS wish to thank the authors, editors, and publishers who granted permission to quote from copyrighted material.

We also wish to thank all the expectant parents who have shared their experiences with us, particularly the members of the original discussion group at the University of California Prenatal Clinic and Shelley and Ben. The material and quotations have been modified to protect the identity of the individuals concerned.

We feel indebted to the many investigators who have contributed to the growing fund of knowledge about the psychology of pregnancy and childbirth and to the many professionals who have earnestly discussed the problems and successes they have experienced in helping families through pregnancy and birth. Special thanks to Sheldon Kopp, who told us we should write this book, and to our editor Justus George Lawler, who actually gave us the opportunity to write it.

We wish to thank our mothers, who were both awake when they brought us into the world and communicated their memories of our births to us as we were growing up. Finally, we want to thank all the people who helped us in pregnancy and childbirth, particularly the obstetricians George Winch and Alan Moss, who delivered our first; Bernard DeVought, who delivered our second; and John Seldon Miller, who delivered our third. All four understood and supported our wish to participate actively in the pregnancy and childbirth experience.

In the twenty years since the publication of the first edition of this book, we have discussed the psychology of pregnancy with hundreds of men and women from all walks of life and varying levels of professional involvement in the field. Our greatest debt is always to the men and women who speak with us so generously about their personal experiences. They remain anonymous, but whenever the words of this book have the ring of truth, it is because of their contributions.

Special thanks are due to Meg Zweibach, R.N., Rohana McLaughlin, M.F.C.C., Pam Krell, Ph.D., Linda Blachman, M.P.H., for discussions relating to current obstetrical care. Gloria Thornton's role as administrator of pregnancy support groups at Mt. Zion Hospital and now at the University of California at San Francisco Medical Center has been instrumental in keeping us involved with women who are currently living the psychological experience of pregnancy. She, like so many other of our colleagues, friends, students, and teachers, is an ongoing source of stimulating conversation about the issues in this book. More particularly, Alicia Lieberman, Ph.D., Kendra Downey, R.N., and Shirley Fischer, C.N.M., read and criticized the manuscript of the revised edition in various stages of development.

Elisabeth Dyssegaard and the editorial staff at The Noonday Press have been exceptionally helpful and competent in the preparation of the revised edition.

We thank them all.

Contents

PREGNANCY
The Psychological Experience

Prologue

WE FIRST BECAME interested in the psychology of pregnancy in 1964, during the nine months before our first child was born. Until then, we had assumed pregnancy was a static condition of little importance apart from its end—labor, birth, the cry of a new baby. When we thought about pregnancy at all, it was as a period of waiting, a non-event. Perhaps we participated in the notion that pregnancy was an indelicate condition that should be kept in the closet and never mentioned in polite society, or that it was a temporary condition best left to the care of obstetricians. We discovered how wrong we had been. Since then, we have devoted a great deal of energy to exploring the emotional and developmental aspects of pregnancy for men and women.

Nine months is too long to write off as a non-experience, to accept as a time of preparation without a reality of its own. A lot happens, both physiologically and psychologically, in that time. Pregnancy is neither a static nor a brief experience, but one full of growth and change, enrichment and challenge. The experience should not be ignored or denigrated; nine months per child might add up to two or even four years in a couple's life, far too long and precious a period to be put in a closet. We decided to look at it more closely. We learned the obvious: that pregnancy is a time full of life and symbolic meaning, change and significance.

Pregnancy is simultaneously a biological, social, and personal transformation that brings one in touch with the archetypal process, that is, with feelings and behaviors and meanings that lie deep within human nature, latent since birth and suddenly evoked by a powerful physical change that reverberates through every other level of the psyche. Pregnancy can be both rewarding and confusing, but at its core it is creative, for at the end there is literally a new life, for the parents as well as for the baby just born.

As we learned more about pregnancy, we realized that a pregnant woman's complaints of anxiety and depression, her frustration with her parents and difficulties with her husband, were part of a special and complex situation. She was a woman enmeshed in a very real change. She didn't need to be "cured" of the emotional upheaval of pregnancy so much as she needed to be guided through expectable dilemmas. She must sort complex new issues in her life and be open to the new identity that is growing within her— not just the identity of the baby, but the identity of herself as a mother, the identity of her partner as a father, and that of her parents as grandparents. With time and experience, we also realized that men were undergoing a psychological transformation similar to that of women. A man is "pregnant" with the role of father growing within him just as his child grows within his partner's womb.

We began to view obstetrical records in a new light. We saw that many pregnancies were described as routine and uncomplicated even when the women became severely depressed after the birth of their children. We wondered how that could be. Could the women really have been stable right up through delivery? Were there no hints of the imminent collapse either in the woman herself or in her partner? Or were medical professionals simply failing to ask the right questions? Perhaps some couples who suspected trouble, and were afraid of what would happen when the baby finally did arrive, were hesitant to describe their anxiety during pregnancy because they did not want to be considered crazy or emotionally unstable. Medical records did not hint at the stress that an anxious couple experienced any more than they reflected the joys of loving couples who were delighted to be creating new life. Yet for both anxious and blissful couples, pregnancy creates an expanding inner world of hope, expectation, fear, and resentment which mirrors the physical reality of the expanding abdomen and growing fetus. Entering the new social roles of parenthood evokes anxiety and challenge, but these charts gave only the physical profile of the mother.

We decided to study pregnancy as a stage in the life cycle. We established a weekly meeting with a group of women who were at the beginning of their first pregnancies. They were normal women, coming to a discussion group at a prenatal clinic because they had been convinced that it might be interesting and significant for them. These women talked about their experiences, their feelings, and their thoughts. They talked of the changes in the way they experienced their bodies, about their new range of sexual feelings, about their husbands, and about their feelings for other people around them. Some of the husbands came to meetings or contacted us informally and became involved in the project. From them we learned how "pregnant" an expectant father could be. Week by week, as their babies grew inside of the women, we heard attitudes and interest change. Gradually, we saw the experience of pregnancy revealed as a pattern of unique psychological states, involving both the woman and her partner in emotions and behaviors they had not known before.

The discussion group continued after the women had given birth. They brought their infants with them. We were surprised to discover that the subject matter moved away from the inner, subjective, experimental themes they had explored when pregnant toward more externally oriented ones, particularly child-rearing. This shift reflected more than just the reality of the new problems associated with the baby. The whole psychological ambience of the women had changed. They were no longer as open to their environment or as responsive to their dreams and fantasies as they had been. They were no longer as likely to respond with extreme sadness to small losses or with overwhelming joy to minor successes. Just as their body silhouettes had slimmed down, so their psychological openness had diminished.

Occasionally we reminded a new mother of something she had said during pregnancy. "That couldn't have been me," she often protested. "It must have been Mary who said that." Even the most psychologically oriented, those who were most willing to investigate the moods and processes of the group, seemed to have lost touch with the condition which they had shared such a short time before. In fact, they rarely wanted to be reminded of the pregnancy experience, except in the form of general, reassuring platitudes.

We wondered how much of the rich emotional material we heard from the women in our group was specific to the first pregnancy, when the changes were new and unfamiliar. Perhaps a couple with another child would already have adapted to the stress of adding a new member; they would already be parents. But we learned that the pregnant woman with children reenters a psychological and physical state familiar to her, with consequences she cannot forget. She is no longer a naïve, first-time mom, but pregnancy is still a demanding change in her life. Anxieties and joys seem to recur with each pregnancy.

Not too surprisingly, after the birth of our first child, we lost interest in pregnancy as well, even though we had tapes and written reports to prove that we had once been enraptured by things that now seemed irrelevant. Our psychological equilibrium had shifted; our child preoccupied us as much as the other infants demanded the attention of their parents. The study produced a paper or two for the psychological literature,[1] but the rest of the notes were filed in the back of a drawer. But when we became pregnant again, the experience, including our acute interest in the inner lives of the pregnant couple, was repeated. Coincident with our third and last pregnancy, we wrote the first edition of this book, which was published in 1971.[2]

We are no longer having babies, and there is a whole new generation working creatively on the subject of pregnancy. We are delighted to see the shelves of libraries and bookstores overflowing with books that prove our point: people are eager to experience pregnancy, childbirth, and parenting as a special and important event in their lives. Why, then, are we revising this old grandparent of a book? Why not leave it to the new generation to describe the experience? Well, we have discovered that there is a place for grandparents. We are no longer inside the experience, but we are still in close contact with men and women who are. As therapists, we see many expectant parents. We are not conducting research of our own anymore, but we often act as consultants to or supervise people who are, and we occasionally conduct a series of interviews with families going through the process, just to stay in touch. We have learned a lot since we first wrote this book, and we have had many requests to bring it up to date. When we would protest that there are so many books on the market now, we were told that our book had a unique point of view because it was willing to expose difficulties without getting lost in negativity and to describe joys without becoming "Pollyannaish." We decided to take on the job of revising and expanding our book, and have incorporated almost twenty years of additional personal and professional experience exploring the psychology of childbearing.

1

The Meaning
of Pregnancy

Cultural attitudes toward pregnant women:
beyond the personal

PREGNANCY HAS ALWAYS been indispensable for human life. No wonder it was the subject of our earliest known artifacts. Archaeologists find statues of large-breasted, big-bellied, fecund women in sites around the world, presumably because pregnancy itself was the object of worship and also because the fertile goddess was considered a powerful deity.

Even though many women experience pregnancy as the apex of their lives, our society does not worship the childbearing woman as the ultimate in feminine power. Her contribution is often denigrated, by women and men alike. Collectively, we have an ambivalent attitude toward reproduction. Some of us fear that there are too many people on the earth already and that our resources may not be enough to go around. Others fear that the world is too unstable or violent for children. Individually, we are also ambivalent. Pregnancy, childbirth, and parenting often distract men and women from their other life goals and drain their emotional and economic resources. For any of these reasons we may choose to avoid getting pregnant or abort a pregnancy that has started.

Modern woman is not the first to be ambivalent about childbearing. Early Egyptian papyri describe contraceptives and give recipes for potions that will stimulate abortion, proving that women in ancient times, like women today, wanted to exert some control over reproduction.

Having a baby has never been considered easy, but it has always been revered as important. When a woman chooses to be fertile and multiply, she enters a realm that goes beyond her personal experience and links her up with the collective. She may at times feel that she is barely clinging to her individual consciousness, the biological imperatives are so overwhelming. She may also feel that other people are seeing their stereotype of pregnancy, not her as a person. She knows she is still herself; she bears the same name and carries the same memories, she comes from the same family and has the same job, but sometimes she feels that she is in the grip of something that is larger than herself, sometimes enhancing her life and sometimes in competition with her "real" self.

A childbearing woman may feel that her body is in the service of the species, that she has become little more than a container for the fetus or a milk machine and comforter for the infant. Pregnancy symbolizes fecundity, nurturance, unconditional love, and creativity. But these concepts are easier to maintain when the pregnancy is happening to someone else; they can overwhelm a woman who is simply trying to deal with her personal life, not carry inspirational meaning for others. Pro-lifers tell her that even an embryo just a few weeks old is more important than she. Doctors probe inside of her, trying to get at the fetus to measure its size or check its chromosomes. Scientists create embryos in test tubes and imply that the womb is an imperfect and temporary vessel for their product. The childbearing woman may feel like an inconvenient adjunct to their work. Is no one taking *her* into consideration?

Every relationship raises the question: Whose needs are more important, yours or mine? Usually there is compromise, creative exchange, and generous interdependency. During pregnancy, one does not get to negotiate the question. The fetus needs the help of the mother to survive, literally needs her lifeblood. The situation is wondrous, but also a little threatening.

A woman discovers that her pregnancy is not only something happening to her personally. It also has meaning to others—and not always a meaning that is compatible with the woman's own inner experience. There are times during the day when a woman in her final month, who is stretching the limits of even her largest maternity dress, forgets that she is pregnant and feels just like herself, an individual with her own private identity. If someone comes along and pats her belly, she is thrust back into the state that she has momentarily forgotten. To the other person she may be the Pregnant Woman. To herself, she is still Mary Jones, and Mary Jones may resent having strangers pat her on the belly or give her unsolicited advice.

Pregnancy places a woman's roles and relationships into a new context, makes her more dependent on a social network for help, and creates intense needs for loving support, attention, and acceptance from others. The way that society views her can profoundly affect her experience, and the possibilities are myriad and unpredictable. Sometimes, pregnant women are perceived as powerful and fertile; other times they are seen as frail, vulnerable, and even sick. A pregnant woman may feel rather like the elephant in the Hindu fable who was groped by the blind men, each of whom came away with an experience of a very different beast. The meaning of pregnancy changes over time even within a culture. In addition, subcultures maintain alternative meanings within a larger society.

Historical overview of modern American attitudes toward reproduction

In the nineteenth century, young America believed in the "procreative imperative." The dominant culture believed in manifest destiny, in their God-given right to populate North America from coast to coast. They needed settlers, and as they developed factories they needed a large labor force and wanted a growing population of consumers for the goods and services being produced in ever greater quantities by American businesses and industries.[1] In her book on the changing views of American motherhood, Maxine Margolis quotes Theodore Roosevelt: " 'If the average family . . . contained but two children, the Nation as a whole would decrease in population so rapidly that in two or three generations it would very deservedly be on the point of extinction. A race that practiced such a doctrine, that is, a race that practiced race suicide, would thereby conclusively show that it was unfit to exist.' "[2]

During the depression of the 1930s, pregnancy was often an extreme financial burden; while values might have been family-oriented, there was not enough food or money to go around. People postponed marriage, unemployed men left wives and children they could not support, and women were overburdened by each new child, no matter how much they loved it. A new pregnancy might threaten the survival of children who had already been born.

After World War II, families were eager to renew and replenish the country. Tired of death and destruction, men and women turned to family life in a peacetime economy. Couples lived out a white-picket-fence fantasy and developed the suburbs. In the 1950s, whole towns consisted entirely of young families, men who left for work each morning and women who stayed at home with their young children. These were the years of the baby boom, the only period in the twentieth century when American women reversed the trend toward having fewer children and having them later. During the fifties, they married younger and gave birth to more babies than in any decade since the nineteenth century.[3]

America of the 1960s has been described as a culture of narcissism.[4] Women of childbearing age found support for remaining child-free; men and women alike began to experiment with new social forms and to take control over their reproductive lives. Nineteen sixty-six, the Summer of Love, and 1969, the Woodstock Festival, epitomize a generation coming of age, moving into adulthood and the childbearing years with sex and drugs and rock and roll. By the 1970s, this new generation had developed a political doctrine that focused on ecological concerns, sexual freedom, women's liberation, and antiracism. Fertility, pregnancy, childbirth, and child care became political topics of great public interest. As people were aware of the dangers of overpopulation, many decided that only one or two children per family was acceptable. A woman hugely pregnant with a third child would have been very uncomfortable walking down the street pushing one child in a stroller and holding another one by the hand. Her fertility became a public issue, not just a personal decision.

Women's liberation emerged as a potent force in the seventies. Feminism's concern for equality moved in two contradictory directions. On the one hand, it heightened awareness of traditionally female tasks such as pregnancy, childbirth, and child care and gave them as much value as traditionally male activities, a position epitomized by the important book *Our Bodies, Ourselves*.[5] On the other hand, feminism insisted (rightfully) that women could be as good as men at traditionally masculine endeavors that required intellect, clarity, energy, and ambition. Unfortunately, this latter emphasis tended to reinforce patriarchal assumptions about the inferiority of traditionally feminine activities and to turn a liberated woman into a pseudo-man rather than a competent and empowered human who also had the ability to bear children. At worst, pregnancy, childbirth, and child care were meaningless activities that should not slow down a "real" woman in her progress through life—that is, in her career.

The meaning of fertility and gender identity in contemporary America

For most women, the reality of ovulation and of possessing a uterus and breasts is incorporated into her positive self-image. The female body is different from the male body. In our male-dominant culture, this often seems a disadvantage and has sometimes been interpreted as making women inferior, but the female body is also often glorified, even held in awe, sought after, admired, and desired. Many women are excited to find that their reproductive body parts function normally.

In some cultures a man's virility may be measured entirely by the number of children he sires, regardless of his sexual competence or the fate of the children. We know of a woman who reported to her doctor that she had not planned one particular pregnancy; she claimed that she had been using several forms of contraceptives at the time of impregnation including the intrauterine device and coitus interruptus. Since she already had eight children at home, this additional one would tax her strength, her health, and her budget. When she was asked how she felt about the pregnancy, she said she was not pleased. When asked how her husband felt, she said, "Well, he may be nuts, but he's as proud as can be."

Fertility is an aspect of female as well as male potency.

We have known women who were not in relationships but who, when they reached their thirties, felt a need to get pregnant just to see whether or not they were fertile. Near the end of their childbearing years, some women become obsessed with having a baby to such an extent that it may impair their ability to concentrate on anything else. The process may be particularly painful for women who aborted earlier pregnancies that occurred at unpropitious times in their lives.

Even in this age of career women who work in the traditional realm of men, conception, pregnancy, and birth remain the domain of women. Like puberty, pregnancy is a time when a person must come up against the dictates of biology. She may or may not be happy with this.

If she values herself primarily as a comrade to men or for her professional activities, pregnancy may be an embarrassment and a real psychological blow. If the relationship between partners is based on complete parity, both sharing equally in work and in domestic responsibilities, the existence of the fetus may force a reevaluation. This may bring the disturbing reminder that there are real role differences between men and women that can be modified but not totally removed by society. A married but childless woman student who was active in the women's liberation movement confided to us in 1970 that she would only have children when her husband understood that all the demands of pregnancy, childbirth, and mothering would be borne equally by him. She might not have achieved total equality, but if she had a baby in the eighties, her partner was probably intensely involved.

In the 1980s, many men became concerned parents from conception on. They were often informed about the medical aspects of pregnancy, participated in childbirth preparation classes, learned about newborn care, sang to the fetus while it was still in the womb, and changed its diapers after it was born. Men did not become the social equals to women in the home—they still lagged behind in performing domestic tasks and assuming the role of primary caregiver for children—but they made great strides toward that goal. Simply the existence of men who acknowledged domestic equality as a goal seemed a revolution to those of us raised during the forties and fifties.

If there is to be a pregnancy, a woman *has* to be involved. A man may or may not be; some cultures surround an expectant mother with women and keep the man away. A "pregnant" man can be seized by an image or a symbol, but his is a much more subjective experience. A pregnant woman's role is dictated by biology. A "pregnant" man can run away from home without finding (as a woman must) that the fetus has come with him, tucked within the womb.

Childbearing may still be some women's most important job, the activity that gives them personal esteem and satisfaction. They may love being pregnant and giving birth and simply want to do it over and over. Some women have religious convictions that encouraged them to fulfill God's commandment to be fruitful and multiply. For others, the continuous childbearing may offer a way to stay dependent on other people, for as long as a woman is pregnant or recuperating from childbirth, she may be free from professional and social pressures to do other things. Most subtly of all, some women are not comfortable as independent adults and prefer to be pregnant or caring for a young baby because it makes them feel whole. They are creating the baby in order to create a mother and to be in the symbiotic relationship that makes them feel more secure.

Many women who wait until their late twenties or early thirties to have a baby experience pregnancy as a rite of passage, the last step in becoming fully adult, fully female. They are often very glad that it takes a full nine months, for they need that time to accommodate to the profound changes that occur. They will soon discover that pregnancy, childbirth, and parenting are more than symbolic events and that, whatever its effect on their development, there is another individual with as much at stake. The child does not exist *for* the mother, even though his or her existence may be gratifying to her. Pregnancy has a profound impact on the mother, but it is a life or death experience for the child.

The impact of the meaning of pregnancy on the child

The circumstances around pregnancy and birth can have a lasting impact on a child's life. We probably all know a family in which one particular child came into the world at an unfortunate time, added an impossible burden, didn't get the security and nurturance he or she needed, and grew up as though blighted—depressed and inconspicuous, feeling unworthy or becoming delinquent, calling for help through misbehavior. For example, we knew a young couple who married in their mid-twenties and had a beautiful and jointly planned first child. When the woman accidentally became pregnant again, the man requested an abortion. She could not imagine terminating the pregnancy and chose to carry the baby, which proved to be an intolerable financial and emotional burden for the family. The mother had less to give, especially to her husband, who turned elsewhere, had an affair during the pregnancy, and missed the birth because he was with his lover. Neither parent ever "fell in love" with the second child the way they had with the first. They both loved it, but the mother was too fatigued, abandoned, depressed, and resentful, the father too preoccupied elsewhere, to nurture an infant fully. The first child remained its parents' comfort and joy, the second a trouble and a problem.

Parents tend to identify with a baby in the same position

of the birth order as they—first child, second, third, etc. Or they may equate a particular pregnancy with a recent loss, and feel that this baby will replace a child or niece or uncle who has just died. One child may become linked with its mother, another with its father. These are the unanalyzable differences between pregnancies. But they do have a real effect on the attitudes toward the pregnancy and toward the child, particularly when it is still in the womb and not asserting its own personality.

The events around the birth itself are often a symbolic statement of a child's meaning in the family. Stories about one's birth are sure to project unconscious feelings about the presence of that person in the family, feelings that are likely to be both positive and negative. In the days of total anesthesia, there might be no family member with a memory of the birth itself. Stories focused on the labor, then a gap, then on seeing the baby ("and you were brought to me . . ."), and on other events surrounding the hospitalization. A child who hears his birth described by his mother, his father, or another family member knows he or she was personally welcomed into the world.

Freudian theory emphasizes the impact of early life experiences on subsequent emotional development. Some people believe that the trauma of birth has permanently scarred us by jarring us from the bliss of the prenatal period and subjecting us to the damaging influence of our parents, particularly our mothers.

The ideal of the "good mother"

All of us, even those who are mothers ourselves, have an image of a perfect nurturer who can care for us and protect us and make us happy, who will not traumatize us but will heal us. Along with this image of the perfect mother for whom we yearn is an opposing image, that of the bad mother who rejected us, failed to protect us, and never loved us enough.

These images of the good and the bad mother convey a difficult message to a pregnant woman: to be a good mother she must take perfect care of her child. She may fear that any negative thoughts she has will damage her child for life; that any trauma in the child's life is her fault. A pregnant woman has an impossible task because the image of the good mother is too good to be true. More realistic theories of child development talk in terms of "good enough" parenting.[6] Parents are imperfect and can only do the best they can.

And yet we yearn for the Madonna, the serene, patient caregiver who devotes all her attention to her child. Even a woman who wants to accomplish important professional goals carries within herself the belief that a mother should protect her infant from all distress, and she wants to be that mother. To accomplish this ideal, the mother herself must be protected within a nest where she can devote herself to gestation, birth, and caregiving. The closer to the birth itself, the more important that a woman be kept safe so that she can bear her child in peace. Other mammals, who ordinarily give birth without trouble, develop problems when the mother is disturbed during labor. Humans, too, although they need the reassuring presence of other people, seem to do best when not distressed by a threatening environment.

Human mothers have a lifetime of experience to add to their minimal repertoire of instinctual behaviors around birth and the care of infants. Infants respond almost entirely from instinct; they have learned only a few things in the womb. They can recognize their mother's voice and are familiar with her body rhythms. They rely almost entirely on the ability of their caregivers to know what they need in the beginning. If a fetus could stay in the womb until twenty-seven months after conception, we could parent more like other mammals, suckle our young for a few weeks or months while they grow steady on their feet and learn to forage for their food. But our infants are born too early in their development, so parents must learn to react in synchrony with any faint traces of instinctual behavior they may feel. Mothers must facilitate labor and birth, relax into lactation, burp a baby properly, and help a newborn learn to self-regulate its states of alertness and sleep. These are the practical aspects of "mother love."

Perhaps the most important factor in determining the ability of a parent to be sensitive to the needs of an infant and to respond selflessly and lovingly is the quality of care that she received as an infant herself.

A new parent's close tie to her infant evokes memories of how it felt to be so connected to her own mother. Unconsciously, a parent repeats her first relationship. For one woman, this may be a warm and wonderful memory. For another, it may be difficult. She may have experienced neglect as well as love. She will want to give more to her own infant than she received herself.

The meaning of merger experiences: "mothered" or "smothered"

Most people are ambivalent about merger experiences because the initial connection with their primary caregiver was both so wonderful and so overwhelming. We are ambivalent both entering into and separating out from the experiences of profound dependency. We are afraid of getting smothered instead of mothered, being held on to rather than held.

In our culture, the Mother, in the abstract, is more often thought of as an adversary than a refuge, especially for men. The smothering mother has been accused of causing everything from school phobia to schizophrenia. Heroic myths include virgins who inspire courage, but the mother figures, usually present in the form of witches and monsters, seek to destroy the hero or render him impotent. Indeed, men who participate in child care, who enter the realm of the mothers, are less likely to be warriors. Nurturance is often experienced as a submerging of individual ambition for the good of others. It is a less self-centered state of consciousness than most and is defined by interconnectedness, not individuality. For some this is its greatest pleasure; for others, its greatest threat.

The nurturing mother is often associated with the earth, as the source of all life and to whose lap we return in death. The legend of Herakles' encounter with a Titan (one of the generation of immortals that preceded the Greek gods) reflects the power of the earth mother. Antaeus was known to be the son of Mother Earth and to be undefeated in battle. The hero Herakles challenged him to battle and soon proved to be the stronger of the two. Again and again, Herakles defeated the Titan, throwing him to the ground. Each time, Antaeus jumped up again, refreshed, seemingly stronger than before. Herakles suddenly realized that Antaeus was receiving new strength from his mother, from Earth herself. Instead of wearing out, he was being renewed each time he touched the earth. Herakles grabbed Antaeus and held him off the ground. Antaeus, cut off from his mother, "withered like an uprooted flower. He died in Herakles's inexorable grip, unable to touch the earth that was the secret source of his strength."[7]

Men are not the only ones ambivalent about depending on the mother. Daughters, too, must make a break, and fear the mother may wish to destroy them rather than let them go. A man must separate from a woman to fulfill his social role. He may have doubts about his masculinity and continue to feel the pull of the "umbilical cord" (or "apron strings"), but he has physical evidence that he is not the same as his mother. A daughter does not necessarily make such a break. She can go from one role in the mother-child dyad to the other without ever experiencing herself as a separate person. If and when she does achieve this separation, she may simultaneously yearn for the comfort of being part of her mother's psyche and fear for the dangers of regressing back into the less conscious state of merger.

Fairy tales such as Snow White mask the fear of the Mother by calling her a stepmother. As the daughter grows up to be more beautiful (more able to attract Prince Charming, more fit to have babies) than the mother, the queen becomes a witch and attempts to kill Snow White. Symbolically, she offers the girl a poison apple, an apparently nutritious item that will make her unconscious, just as an excess of mother-love can render a child unable to move out into the world. It is the prince who saves her, yet inherent in the salvation, in getting married and living happily ever after, is impregnation and becoming a mother, a queen, and a witch herself.

Do we draw strength from our unconscious connection with our original mother when we return, psychologically, to being an extension of her? Or do we become immobilized, infantilized, smothered, and destroyed when we reexperience ourselves as a part of her? The answer depends on the quality of care we received and the way in which we discovered our psychological and emotional autonomy.

Ambivalence toward an intimate connection with the Mother is not just a theme of myths and fairy tales. Real women voice the fear of "becoming like my mother" when they think of having a baby. They are drawn to their identification with her even when they have rejected her style, but they fear that they will become the wicked witch and have feelings of rage toward their own children.

Toward separation and individuation

Becoming a parent is a process of continuing the cycle. During pregnancy, a woman is mother and child in one physical entity; and yet the mother is always custodian of her own consciousness and the fetus is always developing toward separation and increasing individuation.

Cultures that worship fertility goddesses often include the relationship between mother and daughter in their mysteries. In the myth of Demeter and Persephone, masculine violence disrupts the bond between mother and daughter. Persephone, the daughter, is raped and abducted by Pluto and carried off to become queen in a new realm. But the mother cannot bear the separation, and finally convinces Zeus to let Persephone return to her. When her daughter arrives, Demeter rouses from her depression and the earth springs into bloom. When Persephone returns to her husband, Demeter's depression results in the withering of crops, in the arrival of winter. Demeter is a mother who cannot bear to let her child go; Persephone is a daughter who can only be powerful in her own right when she gets away from her mother.

Every mother becomes like Demeter when she gives birth to children who will some day be torn from her (even when they skip away happily on their own, the separation may feel like a violation to the mother). In the natural development of parenting, a mother (and if he is involved as a nurturer, the father) moves from an almost total union of parent and child, one body undifferentiated from the other, to a new mother with a babe in arms, to a woman holding a squirming child in her lap, to a parent who watches as her child moves out into the yard, the school, the nation, and the world. Sooner or later she must let go, must watch her daughter run off with Prince Charming or Pluto, or see her son meet a seductress or the girl next door.

Many men and some women go through childbearing and -rearing without entering a state of merger, of blurred boundaries and identity confusion. They may be less likely to experience the depression of separation, and perhaps also less likely to feel some of the positive sensations of intimate nurturing. Most mothers and fathers get caught in the profound connection between parent and child to a greater or lesser degree. Giving one's self over to this experience may feel to some like a psychic death, but the process of contact with the Great Mother can, as for Antaeus, renew, strengthen, and enrich. We think of the experience as resembling orgasm in the sense that one lets go, enters totally beyond consciousness into the biological/personal/spiritual moment, and then emerges as consciousness reassembles and life goes on.

To be defined in part by our close relationship to others need not restrict or confine our identity. The personal self is in relation to the other, not taken over entirely by the other. There may be moments when the parent's personal identity seems overwhelmed, but those moments also enhance her ability to encompass a multitude of states and live life fully. Just as she must tolerate times of intense connectedness, so, too, a new parent must tolerate times of acute separation. Sometimes she may feel as though a limb has been amputated when she is apart from her child, and yet the baby must develop inexorably toward independence. A "good enough" parent may experience both extremes. Allowing the vulnerability of the moment does not render her unable to function, but frees her to live out all the roles of the life cycle.

2

The Expectant Mother's Experience

EACH PREGNANCY is unique. Every woman reacts to the fairly predictable physiological sequence in her own way. The same woman may react differently to each successive pregnancy. Nevertheless, there is a certain quality of inner experience that seems to be distinctive of the pregnant state and which sets it slightly apart from life at any other time and which every woman encounters to some degree. These are the archetypal aspects of pregnancy, the mysterious combination of biological and social factors that seem to be released sequentially as we move through the life cycle and that subtly influence our development from one stage to another.

Universally, women experience pregnancy as a psychological as well as a physical event. It could not be otherwise. Shifts in body image, secretions of hormones, and the maze of changing environmental supports and cultural expectations are inevitably mirrored in the psyche, in the mental life of the pregnant woman. Changes in identity go hand in hand with changes in body and role. The process may be smooth or violent, reassuring or frightening, happy or sad, but it is certainly change.

Any period of such profound transformation can be called a "crisis."[1] When psychologists and sociologists use the word, they do not mean anything terrible, only that events that may seem routine to the people going through them are actually of greater significance than usual. Even when a pregnant woman feels that she is just going about her business, she is also participating in a larger event that is inexorably shaping her future. She is concentrating on the events of the moment, but when they pass, her life will never be the same again.

A pregnant woman may not seem very different to the casual observer, and she may not admit to feeling very different, but she has embarked on a journey through tremendous internal and external change that sometimes leads to social and personal transformation. As with other gradually occurring phenomena, the pregnant woman may recognize shifts in her emotional reactions or perceptual world only when they begin to affect others—perhaps her husband or her other children—who then call them to her attention. She may cry more easily at movies, react more strongly to a trivial event in her domestic life, become prone to sudden bouts of anxiety with little apparent reason, switch more rapidly from anger to forgiveness, or be moved more readily to profound states of aesthetic appreciation than would be characteristic of her in her nonpregnant state. Technically, this is known as "emotional lability," a psychological condition characterized by a wide range of rapidly shifting moods in response to situations that would not generally trigger such reactions. The pregnant woman's emotional highs and lows are often of greater magnitude than usual for her. They may come and go more quickly, and pass through extremes at a pace that can be confusing and distressing to herself and to those close to her.

Gradually, as the world about her responds to the pregnant woman's slightly unusual reactions, she will become aware of her altered emotional state. She may overreact to apparently neutral events and begin to reflect upon the cause. She may find no objective reason for her outbursts and mood changes. But even when a simple or profound one is discovered, it may not help. Her lability may continue.

Pregnant women may become terribly anxious or depressed, burst into tears or uncontrollable laughter during small family arguments. They may suddenly be unable to make simple decisions or be frightened by a stranger on the street whose face seems to haunt them. One woman consistently became upset when she received or was afraid she might receive the wrong change at a store. And a few of the women in the clinic discussion group stopped going out with friends because they were embarrassed at their own inappropriate and extreme outbursts in public.

This emotional lability will be more pronounced in some women than in others, depending on their personality structure, the kind of real stress they are under, and the quality of actual support they receive. It is also likely that hormonal changes play an important role and may be very different in one pregnancy than in another.

All pregnant women participate in this altered emotional state to some extent, though many seem unaware of it. The obstetrical literature is filled with experimental and clinical data describing and measuring anxiety, insomnia, crying spells, and so forth. For example, one obstetrician found that "the blues" were described by 84 percent of pregnant women, compared to 26 percent of nonpregnant women in a control group. "Unexplained crying" was described by 68 percent of the pregnant women compared to 5 percent of the control group.[2] Another research group found that 50 percent of their normal clinic population reported that they were anxious, experienced emotional lability, and had difficulty sleeping while they were pregnant.[3] Psychological testing of matched pregnant and nonpregnant groups and in the same individuals during and after pregnancy has shown similar increases in anxiety, depression, and, surprisingly, the number of errors in test of cognitive function.[4] When professionals in the mental health field evaluated such clinical and experimental findings in the past, they interpreted them as indicating some kind of emotional pathology. Their judgment should probably be modified in the case of pregnant women. The following is a clinical description of a woman who, in her nonpregnant state, appeared to be quite normal:

> She gives a number of responses that suggest a breakdown of ego controls. She tends to react in a very flat way emotionally, evidently withdrawing to some extent from the world around her. There is a tendency to paranoid thoughts at times, especially in the more distressing situations when her controls break down. It is hard to know whether she is really psychotic, pre-psychotic, disorganized, or *simply pregnant.*[5]

Six months after she gave birth to her child, this woman came across as "pleased and relaxed about her situation." She had, apparently, been "simply pregnant." Perhaps it would be more accurate to say that she had been "complexly pregnant."

As with other life crises, pregnancy creates a delicate balance between positive and negative experiences, between growth and regression. Every moment of joy, anticipation, creativity, and exhilaration is likely to be balanced by one of anxiety, ambivalence, loss, and fear. Although there are emotional problems in pregnancy, most are rooted in the normal reactions to change and development. But it can be difficult to see them as normal when one is in the middle of them.

Some people try to limit the extent of their involvement in the pregnancy experience, including its strange feelings and fantasies, because they are afraid of psychological damage, either to themselves or to the fetus. There is little rationale for these feelings; severe emotional problems during pregnancy are rare. We even suspect that the women who are most fully aware of the changes of pregnancy have less trouble adjusting after the baby is born. They will not fall prey to the "sunny pregnancy syndrome," the situation of a woman who breezes through pregnancy acknowledging only positive and optimistic feelings and then finds herself plummeted into despair after the baby is born. She has an unrealistic view of childbirth, infants, and herself and has not done the psychological "work" of pregnancy. She has not used the time to readjust her inner and outer life to the changes that come with parenthood. The emotional upheaval in pregnancy can be an appropriate and adaptive reaction to life events.

If biological processes, body changes, and parenthood are not very important to a woman, she will keep the pregnancy at a greater distance from her consciousness. One study suggests that "a woman who denies or rejects her body will find pregnancy and motherhood difficult and conflicting."[6] One way of dealing with this is to parent from a distance, a pattern that is easier for a man but also common among women. Throughout the ages wealthy mothers have handed their babies over to other women—wet nurses or nannies— as soon as they emerge. At the opposite end of the socioeconomic scale, poor women have also frequently had to give their babies to others to take care of. They need to work outside the home to support their children (ironically, wet nurses were often poor women who had to abandon their own infants to care for those of others). A woman who returns to work immediately (and we have heard stories of women who bring the nanny with them to the hospital, hand over the baby on the spot, and return to the office) has less need to go through a personal transformation on becoming a mother. She accepts her infant as a responsibility added on to her already complex life, and she may be fully competent to manage the task and provide an appropriate primary caregiver. Traditional wealthy Chinese families hired an *Ima* (nanny) for each new baby. The servant became the child's devoted nurturer for the rest of her life while the mother was left free to play a more supervisory role in the family's life.

Each of the members of the pregnancy study group was afraid at one time or another that her mind was slipping. She usually brought the matter up as a joke, lightly describing a fear or an obsession, and only gradually admitting how truly frightened and worried she had been about her own emotional health. Sometimes the whole group talked about insanity, reassuring each other and laughing nervously about their strange dreams and thoughts. Insanity is a universal fear, only barely hidden by the stability of routine adjustment. At times of personal crisis, such as pregnancy, when the familiar patterns have to be changed, we are more vulnerable to fears of the unknown and of the irrational. Talking about them seems to help make them more understandable.

Pregnancy seems to provide its own counterbalancing protection against mental breakdown. One study demonstrates that pregnant women commit suicide only one-sixth as often as nonpregnant women in comparable age groups.[7] Before legalized abortion, suicide *attempts* occurred among pregnant teenagers, but even here the cry for help seems more important than a real desire to kill oneself.[8] With legal abortions and improved birth control, this once-desperate situation for young women has altered dramatically, although birth control and abortion are still issues of serious concern to childbearing women, as we will discuss in our section on the first trimester of pregnancy.

Perhaps because pregnancy is always a time-limited condition, people are willing to wait and see whether emotional distress will pass instead of going for psychiatric help. Whatever the reasons, medical mythology holds that pregnancy is a time when a woman is less susceptible to severe mental disease, just as the premenstrual days and menopause are held to be the times of highest risk.

When asked "How do you feel?" or "What is your mood like?" the pregnant woman may be able to answer only for a given day, or even a given hour, knowing from prior experience that she is likely to feel very different soon. Unless she is very sure about the attitudes and the patience of her listener, she may try to give a bland answer, rather than distress or embarrass her nonpregnant questioner with the truth. Time and again during prenatal checkups, a pregnant woman talks about what she thinks *the doctor* will want to listen to. The problem, then, is to whom can she turn? Her husband is in the throes of his own conflicts. Women who have made confidantes of their mothers may now find themselves more competitive, less dependent, and afraid of being misled by the outmoded advice of a previous generation. Other pregnant women and new mothers may take on a new significance, as the only people who can really empathize, share opinions, and give advice. Friends and social support are particularly important in a time of such rapid change and confusing choices.

On the other hand, if anyone really shows genuine interest in hearing more than a perfunctory "fine" or "okay," the pregnant woman will almost certainly be extraordinarily eager to describe her feelings in greater detail than she ordinarily would. Repeatedly, studies have shown that pregnant women are far more open and more willing to spill forth dreams, fantasies, anxieties, and pleasures—all highly personal—than normal individuals in nonpregnant states. They are interested in and want to describe the minutiae of their psychological condition, as though every chance to talk about it is a chance to explore and master the experience.

This willingness of pregnant women to talk personally to others about their uncanny experiences is an expression of the universal need for an explanation of the unknown. Some of the more psychologically oriented members in the discussion group ruminated about possible reasons for a particularly bizarre fantasy, pervasive dream, or ecstatic moment. Sometimes group discussions were able to isolate a particular bit of personal history or a psychological mechanism that might have been responsible for the fantasies or feelings of the day. Others, afraid to delve into the mysteries of the mind in a time of stress, sought alternative systems of explanation. One of the most popular and comforting of these was the pseudo-medical rationale that hormonal changes were entirely responsible for their mood swings and unexplained anxieties.

Scientific findings show that the hormonal shifts of pregnancy do have an impact on the emotional swings of the mother. Progesterone, estrogen, corticosteroids, and other hormones involved in the hormonal changes of pregnancy are thought to have some effect in mediating emotions, particularly depression and elation. That is not to say that they *create* emotions or that they have any influence on the content of emotions. Humans are too complex for any such simple explanation. The pregnant woman is living with an altered internal chemical environment which, in interaction with all the other physical, environmental, and cultural factors, will be part of the pregnancy experience. Hormones do not alter the feeling state in a direct way that is consistent for all women. They may influence the intensity of a feeling, but its quality and content depend on the context, on the pregnant woman's inner and outer life.

Whatever the current explanation for psychological changes during pregnancy, at some time during the nine months most women experience these changes as alien and even dangerous. Some think they are "going crazy" when they burst into tears without warning or become afraid in situations where they used to feel secure. Usually they can laugh sheepishly at themselves a day or two afterward, when their thoughts and emotions have turned in more positive directions. More particularly, they often believe that their mood changes and other unusual psychological states might have a lasting influence on the baby. This fear is a modern counterpart to widely held folk superstitions in which people believe that what the pregnant woman sees or hears, thinks or does will directly affect the baby's development and the course of its life. Most Americans now consider such magical thinking bizarre and primitive, but similar concepts may occur even to a modern, sophisticated mother-to-be. She may spend hours listening to classical music or staring at paintings in a museum, hoping to create a great artist or, at the very least, a peaceful disposition in her child. Or she may be afraid to visit a zoo or to be in the same room with a parrot because the beak or trunk of a bird or beast might affect the physiognomy of the unborn baby.

Medical science partially supports this ancient superstition by providing evidence of the ways that a pregnant woman's behavior can affect the fetus. Most blatant are cases of fetal drug addiction, fetal alcohol syndrome, and fetal AIDS infection, cases in which the baby's physical condition is profoundly affected by the mother's behavior. Less discernible are cases in which a baby's birth weight and/or health may have been impaired by caffeine, nicotine, aspirin, or other substances ingested by the mother.

We are just beginning to learn about the subtle ways in

which a fetus is influenced by its mother's moods and behavior. We know that anything that causes the mother's circulatory system to contract will impede the flow of blood to the placenta and deprive the fetus of oxygen, at least momentarily. For example, chronic stress may create a situation of chronic oxygen deprivation, which in turn retards fetal growth, but the evidence indicates that this only occurs in extreme situations.[9] Normal variations in blood flow, caused by expectable fluctuations in the mother's levels of stress, are thought to create normal changes, to which the fetus can adjust.

In recent years studies have shown that definite learning goes on in the womb.[10] A newborn prefers his mother's voice to all others. He also prefers to hear his mother read stories that she read aloud in the last weeks of pregnancy. The baby is "present" in the family before it is born and is subtly influenced by the environment, the voices, music, and moods that surround it. But we cannot be more specific about the influence of events or the mother's moods on the developing baby. A fetus does not understand language or "know" people; it simply grows familiar with its environment and prefers the familiar to the strange.

One woman in our discussion group said:

> I know when women get pregnant they sometimes, you know, the feeling changes and I don't want to be . . . I don't want it to have an effect on my child . . . well, you're supposed to stay calm, anyway, and the more strain you put on all your processes is supposed to—may not be harmful, but is certainly not beneficial.

The woman was afraid that her tensions and anxieties might communicate themselves to the baby and influence not just its health but its future attitudes. Thus she tried to control her mood swings so that only "good" ones, such as concern for her husband's safety, might be experienced.

It is highly unlikely, however, that anything as simple as "bad thoughts" can have an adverse effect on the baby. Thoughts do not transfer to the baby's mind even though it is living inside the mother's body. The communication occurs in two ways: through the chemicals that pass from the mother's blood to the baby's through the placenta, and through hearing and touch as those senses develop and are perceived in the fetal brain. The fetus also develops the ability to see and taste and smell, but it is harder to communicate to a child through these senses while it is living inside the womb unless one initiates a conscious and elaborate procedure.

Most babies seem to respond with vigor to the fluctuation of mood, stress level, anger, frustration, and happiness of the typical woman living through a normal pregnancy. Perhaps they even benefit from exposure to such a range of experiences, for these are the conditions into which they will be born. We have seen women refuse to acknowledge problems in their marriages or in their living arrangements because they did not want to have any "bad," that is, angry, feelings during the pregnancy. Surely the baby would benefit from having a mother who could confront her feelings and take responsibility for her life circumstances. Life is not free from conflict. Repressing negative thoughts and feelings does not protect the fetus.

Nevertheless, women who are concerned about protecting their unborn babies from unnecessary stress are being good and appropriate parents. Cultures that value children highly are particularly apt to caution women that they must modify their lives to protect the vulnerable baby. An American woman who bore a child in Japan described her experience there:

When I announced my pregnancy, it was assumed that I would quit my teaching position and drop out of language school. My teacher told me that language study was stressful, and the increased levels of epinephrine that it caused were harmful to the baby. Similarly, I was advised that the noise of train travel, typing, or using a sewing machine should be avoided.[11]

Current values in the United States are much more likely to support a woman's desire to continue working, traveling, and participating in her usual activities without any suggestion that the fetus will suffer. On the contrary, many women feel that vigorous exercise or loud music will stimulate their developing child in positive ways. Our culture may be more afraid of the bad influence of an overprotective mother than that of an overactive mother.

While specific subjects, thoughts, or words cannot be communicated to the fetus, they often do trigger extreme emotions in a normal pregnant woman. The baby is having a powerful impact on her; it is less clear what kind of impact she is having on the baby. A magazine picture of a contented, healthy baby may call forth an intense response—as the advertising industry knows well. Pregnant women may be particularly susceptible to war pictures, or to posters showing starving children. Members of a support group in 1988 agreed that they had been most moved by the movie *Gorillas in the Mist* and by a news story of stranded whales.

Our sense of the infant's extreme vulnerability is an understandable and even fortunate part of our evolutionary history, since our babies are born so immature and in need of protection. Our sensitivity to the awesome responsibility of parenthood was displayed on many car windows in the late 1980s through bright yellow signs that read BABY ON BOARD, as though the parents expected everyone to drive differently because of their precious burden. The same profound, virtually biological, impulse to protect babies is present in people's solicitous attitude toward pregnant women. Dynamic businesswomen often prefer to dress to conceal their pregnancies because they are uncomfortable with this response from men they consider their competitors, peers, or subordinates, not their protectors.

One woman in our original discussion group read a Catholic weekly newspaper which often carried editorials condemning people who were in favor of birth control and abortion. She recognized early in her pregnancy that she felt uneasy whenever she read these editorials, but by the sixth or seventh month, such material reduced her to tears. During the last month of her pregnancy, she was unable to read about a fetus without becoming tearful and depressed. Her overreaction was probably affected by her own attitudes and situation. She acknowledged that she had not wanted to become pregnant and wished she were not having a baby.

The topics of death and dying hold a continual fascination for the pregnant woman. A newspaper account of the accidental death of some children triggered a long, ruminating discussion in the group, and the discussion continued compulsively, even though it was upsetting. It was as if, by being closer to birth, to the beginning of life, pregnant women were automatically closer to death. In fact, pregnant women are more in touch with their entire life cycles than at other times. Death, maiming, and injury are inescapable possibilities in their situation. Perhaps the need to talk about death is an attempt to achieve a psychological mastery over this vulnerability. As one woman in the discussion group put it, "You're just thinking more about life and death, and not wanting to be hurt in any way, you know, that would harm the child. I think it's a natural thing." The others agreed with her. This association between birth and death is sometimes a motive for the pregnancy itself. Women often decide, consciously or unconsciously, to create a new life when they have suffered the loss of someone they love dearly. Women seem particularly likely to become pregnant in the early months after the death of their father, as though to become a part of the stream of life.

The willingness of pregnant women to talk about their

experiences is often surprising, particularly to men, who tend to think of pregnancy as a withdrawn, inner state that cannot be shared. And to a great extent this is true. If not encouraged to share, a pregnant woman might sit silently, knitting and rocking or staring poignantly out the window. She may seem more in touch with things, more easily gratified by working with her hands. Pregnant women often take up a creative hobby, such as painting or gardening. Sewing and knitting are traditional interests which are not only appropriate to the creative impulse and to the soft, quiet mood, but also have particular value in helping a woman focus on the reality of her changing figure as she makes maternity clothes, and on the imminence of the baby as she prepares a layette. Time spent knitting baby clothes feels to her like time spent caring for the unborn baby.

A woman has not necessarily gone blank when she falls silent or lets herself float along in a fog. She is, so to speak, sitting next to the flow of life, close to its source. If one induces her to talk, she is likely to be able to describe the experience in detail. Even her language is enriched. Commonplace words have become fuller and more significant, carrying new life, like the woman herself. Everyday phrases such as "I conceived an idea," "the statement was pregnant with meaning," "I will bear it in mind" become concrete expressions. Less transparent words like "full," "seed," "egg," or "fruitful" take on extra weight. The woman might pause as she speaks, realizing suddenly why she chose to express herself as she did. Just as likely, she will never notice the relationship between her condition and her language. If she talks of a "refrigerator so full it could almost burst," she might or might not realize that she is obliquely talking about herself.

Words like "kicking" and "pounding" take on new, more internal meanings as women experience these things from a new aspect, more intimately and concretely. Metaphor and fact are fused in a rare and wonderful way. "Seeds," "fertility," and "birth" are no longer objective terms. On some days, even a word like "fish" may be a psychological concept rather than a neutral word. "No, I am not strong enough to go to the zoo today. I want to go to the aquarium and watch the big fish. Some of them are even big enough to eat other fish." In this case, the fish may suggest the fetus in the uterus and also, perhaps, recall Jonah who lived in the whale. Women often describe the movement of the fetus early in the pregnancy as a "fishy" feeling and imagine the womb as a vessel filled with water. The idea of another creature living inside one's body can be difficult to grasp!

The word "explosion" may no longer suggest to a woman the idea of something external "going off" and sending forth flying splinters and thus destroying things. Rather, it is likely to be experienced as something inside "blowing up." A totally neutral picture, as in a psychological test, may be transformed into a parable for a woman's own feelings about her condition. One pregnant woman kept interpreting things as getting worse; she kept thinking of raging fires which were getting out of control or balloons that were getting bigger and bigger until they might pop. For her, the fetus was a kind of time bomb.

Sudden compulsive urges to do a thorough housecleaning seem common among pregnant women. They are, on one level, practical attempts to prepare for the coming baby; but when the house is already amply clean and delivery is impending, there may be a second, more significant meaning. The woman may be acting out her unconscious identification of the house with her own body. She may feel that if she cleans out the house and puts everything in order, she is in some way doing something about that other living space, the "house" of her unborn child. For her, it is an object rather than a word, which has taken on secret meanings. Women have been known to feel particularly close to ripe fruit, as they identify with their own seed and with the fruit of their womb. A woman may feel that she has entered the Garden of Eden as she sits beneath a large, leafy tree and eats its swollen, seedy fruit, for she is closer to the primal experience of mankind than at other times. More mundane things can also become meaningful. A tight squeeze through a narrow passage may bring a nervous giggle which seems, at first, related only to the unexpected difficulty arising from her enlarged figure. If examined further, however, there are more subtle innuendoes for the woman soon to be delivered. She is identifying with the fetus.

Women are less likely to describe themselves as looking like blimps than like whales or ripe watermelons. That is, they identify with swollen objects that bear life rather than with those that are merely round and empty. As a pregnant woman becomes increasingly aware of the changes taking place inside her body, she is likely to identify with physical objects that are similar to her feelings about herself. She may feel as though she were a part of the refrigerator she is using or the house she is living in. She may identify with a goldfish bowl, both in shape and contents but also in feeling exposed and stared at. One woman talked about her new home, which had a bay window: "It is as though the whole house is full and pregnant and warm," she said.

Pregnant women may feel irrationally attracted or repelled by certain otherwise insignificant objects. Some may suddenly worry about "eggs" which they have heard may create a "bad reaction" if eaten by pregnant women. Others are just as likely to make sure to eat an egg a day, feeling that this is a critical nutritional asset.

Food and the act of ingestion acquire special meanings and may become a many-faceted symbol during pregnancy.

Gaining weight early in the pregnancy may serve as a kind of proof that the baby, still invisible, is growing. A woman who very much wants to be pregnant and to have a baby may put on ten pounds in the first three months, so great is her enthusiasm at the prospect of displaying to the world and to herself her wonderful condition. Even slight attacks of nausea will not dampen her eagerness to take things into her body and make it grow. She may be able to reduce her intake after about the sixth month, when her uterus itself becomes large enough to be visible through her clothing.

A woman may discover that her weight is an aspect of pregnancy that she *can* control. By overeating, a woman can feel she is contributing to the growth of her abdomen instead of being a passive observer in nature's grand scheme. But our cultural obsession with thinness also influences a woman's experience of pregnancy. A woman whose figure is important to her self-esteem may have trouble incorporating her new breasts and belly and may feel (especially in the first half of the pregnancy) that her extra inches are "fat." Some women refuse to go swimming during pregnancy because they are ashamed of their bodies. Undereating can be as important a form of control for one woman as overeating is for another.

Children often assume that the mouth, rather than the vagina, is the portal through which a baby passes to enter the mother's body. They may think that it emerges through the anus. This distorted idea of conception and delivery sometimes becomes extreme, even pathological, and may carry into adulthood. Women who are ignorant about their bodies may think that anything that goes in through the vagina could get forced up into the throat. Misconceptions of this kind can cause fear and confusion. Freudian theory suggests that a woman might refuse to eat and become anorexic because of a fear of being orally impregnated. Recent studies indicate that this fear of impregnation is rare but that some anorexics may fear being invaded by another person. Pregnancy will be emotionally threatening to a woman with such concerns, for in this state there actually is one human being living inside another. [12]

Many women are reassured to discover there are things they can do to affect the course of the pregnancy or the development of the fetus. The influence of a proper diet is obvious: the proper amount of iron will affect a woman's energy level; calcium will eliminate leg cramps. These factors are evident to a woman who has a problem and sees it disappear by taking a pill. She may then move into less precise areas of influence, such as switching to a high-protein diet to help the baby's brain develop or taking an extra vitamin to encourage a particular trait. In fact, women who take vitamins around the time of conception and in the early months of pregnancy are decreasing their risk of giving birth to a baby with certain kinds of serious deformities. At the extreme, a woman may become a vegetarian in order to eliminate violence from her child, or she may eat only natural, unprocessed food so that the child will remain uninfluenced by "the establishment." She may also be extra careful about additives and preservatives because of her concern that even small doses of chemicals that might be safe for adults may be harmful to the delicate formation of the body of the fetus. The warning labels on alcoholic beverage containers and the signs on restaurant walls reminding consumers that the ingestion of alcohol by pregnant women may affect the health of the fetus are constant reminders to expectant mothers of the power of their behavior to shape their child's future.

Many old traditions about the role of food in pregnancy may also affect a woman's reaction to her food. Innumerable jokes base their humor on the cravings of pregnant women, mocking her but also freeing her to be eccentric. The stories of women who crave pickles and ice cream and men who go out into the storm at night to get them legitimize the possibility that women may have irrational whims and that men may be expected to satisfy them during this time.

The fairy tale of Rapunzel addresses a darker side of women's cravings during pregnancy. "Once there was a woman who wanted to have a little child more than everything else in the world," the story begins.[13] As in the pregnancy dreams of real women and in many other fairy tales, the woman gets pregnant with the baby that she so desired, but then she loses it to the wicked witch. Once she is pregnant, her craving for food supersedes her craving for the baby:

> Now the wife liked to sit and look from her upstairs window into the garden next door. It belonged to a witch, and all sorts of wonderful flowers and vegetables grew there. One day the wife noticed a patch of salad greens. These looked so crisp and delicious that the woman's mouth watered for them. The more she gazed on the shining green leaves the more her longing for them increased until she grew sick and weak, and her husband feared she would die if she could not have some of the witch's salad greens. So one evening he climbed over the garden wall to get some for her.[14]

This husband was too indulgent of his wife's desires; the salad greens he stole were called "rapunzel." When the wicked witch discovered what he had done, she stole the baby as soon as it was born and named it Rapunzel.

This fairy tale touches two themes of pregnancy (not to mention the virtually universal theme of childhood, that "I can't be the true child of this wicked witch who is raising me"). First, it demonstrates that a baby may be profoundly affected by what its mother eats and even what she thinks. If the mother had not seen or thought about or eaten the rapunzel, the family could have lived together happily forever after. Second, it suggests that the husband has to use his judgment when he tries to make his wife happy. At the center of the story is the age-old problem of establishing whose needs come first. When only one can be satisfied, it suggests, the mother may have to deprive herself for the well-being of her child. This mother, who thought she would have done anything for her child, progresses to a stage where she would have done anything to get her rapunzel; her concern is more with having her whim satisfied than with being a parent.

While "Rapunzel" is a cautionary tale, the demands and needs of pregnant women are very serious indeed. Any particular desire may seem silly or self-indulgent, but the issue is profound. Human infants need to be cared for by a loving adult. That adult is usually the mother, who is faced with her own growing dependency needs. She cannot do the job well in isolation. Late in pregnancy, certainly during the birth itself, and for the early months of infancy, a mother needs protection; she is encumbered by her child and by her biological process. Every time she feels an urge for pickles or ice cream, she is really testing other caregivers in her life. Is there anyone in the family who will take care of her without question? The survival of our species has been based on the answer to that question. Every woman should ask it, one way or another. Good prenatal medical care includes an assessment of the woman's support system: who will go for pickles and ice cream, or rather, who will give the woman love and affection during pregnancy, attention and care during labor and birth, and practical as well as emotional help in the postpartum period? The husband is often expected to fill all these roles.

Car phobia is a particularly common theme of pregnancy. It may come on quite suddenly, usually after the first motions of the fetus have been felt. The car becomes an extension of the woman's own body and therefore much more at risk than usual. But her concern often focuses on her husband's driving. The women in our original group discussed this issue at length. They realized that they were afraid of being abandoned after the baby was born. Many had fears that their husbands might die and they would have to take care of the child alone. One woman spoke about her husband's driving; the others focused intensely on every word, as though she were speaking for them all:

> I'm more concerned with my husband's driving too. He's not the safest driver. It's never bothered me before but now coming off the freeway you know [Oh boy! You too?] I was about hanging on to the edge of the chair and went "Hmmmm haaa aaah!" and then I'd say excuse me, because going "haah"—you know—is going to upset him while he's driving a car, but I can't help it—it looks like we're going to hit everything in sight. [I know what you mean!] You know—and he passes too far to the right and you know I'm hanging on to the door! Well, it is sort of an annoying and a little bit of a nerve-racking thing, but not the way I've been taking it lately. I just know we're going to hit something. I can't conceive of us really dying, but I know we're going to hit something. And then it's going to be too late . . .

The increased vulnerability undoubtedly relates to fear of unknown dangers, both inside and out. A woman no longer knows her own body and she has lost the sense of how she appears to others. Even the hard realities of the freeway become frightening unknowns. She must rely on someone else to steer her way through life, and she is not sure whether or not she can trust her partner. Will he keep her safe? Will it get out of control? These are very important questions for the pregnant woman to address.

Physical symptoms of pregnancy express a woman's deep anxiety about her state. Occasionally, a specific emotional difficulty is expressed through a particular physical symptom such as nausea or a headache. More often, an array of changing medical concerns reflects a persistent psychological theme. For example, one woman experienced the first half of her pregnancy as idyllic. As soon as her baby began to move, however, she seemed less euphoric. She started to talk about vague abdominal problems, and, simultaneously, about how inadequate her own mother had been when she was a child. She became less sure that childbirth would be a marvelous experience. She began to worry about the baby's position in her uterus, and became afraid that her baby would develop a blood disease. Reassurance helped only for a little while. She was sure something would go wrong. She dreamed about terrible accidents to the child. She finally announced, in the ninth month, that she had a "broken sacral vertebra." She was so sure that she insisted her doctor take an X ray. When the results came back she would not believe them. She was sure her sacral vertebra was broken. Her anxiety grew more intense as labor drew closer. Finally she gave birth to a healthy baby; her fears were forgotten and her symptoms disappeared. She had been expressing all her emotional conflicts as medical problems. She was extremely afraid of giving birth and wanted to prove that she had a physical problem that would make it impossible. Fortunately, she had a family and a medical staff that were willing to be patient and continue to reassure her throughout the process. They kept reminding her that it only *felt like* she had a broken sacral vertebra and that it *felt like* she could not survive, but that, in fact, her body was fine. Her fears were real, but they were focused on false issues. As she was told over and over that her body was fine and could do the job, she did succeed in relaxing into the natural process of labor and gave birth normally.

The pregnant woman is in close touch with her inner world. Unconscious processes are much closer to the surface and more available to her than at most times in the life cycle. Her fantasies and dreams provide some of the most dramatic evidence of the changes in her psychology. It is probably not that she actually dreams more, since dream research suggests that we each dream in a consistent pattern every night. Rather, dreams and daytime fantasies seem to be experienced more immediately and intensely during pregnancy. The outer world becomes relatively less important and the inner world relatively more important. Dreams seem to invade the imagination as the fetus occupies the abdomen.[15] Women are reported in various studies as having dreams that seemed as real and as intense as anything that happened during the day. One woman described her dream as pursuing her into the day and affecting her more personally than any she had had before she was pregnant. She was echoed by another woman who described her need to "go around all day trying to get it off my mind . . . getting a book and reading it to keep from concentrating on the dream."

The increased importance of obsessions, phobias, and dreams may be embarrassing and alien to a pregnant woman, and such matters are generally brought up only with some hesitation. In the discussion group, however, the other women always responded with shared emotions and relieved feelings. Perhaps the most memorable moments in the group were those occasions when one of the women would mention a "peculiar thought" that she was having, or the particularly frightening dream that she had had "a month ago," and then the other women, to the obvious relief of them all, would admit to similar experiences. Some women seemed able to give themselves over to the dreams and fantasies, not as an escape, but as a way of capturing the potential richness of their new inner life.

As the power and intensity of women's dreams and inner life are affected by their pregnant state, so too is the content of their dreams. One investigator reports that 40 percent of the dreams described by the pregnant women he studied were about a baby, compared to only 1 percent of the dreams of college women in the same age range.[16] Pregnant women also dream more frequently about misfortunes, harm, and environmental threats.

Misfortune dreams are frequently about the dreamer herself being trapped or in grave danger:

> MARY: I feel some terrible harm is going to come to me and it's specific. It's not some unknown shadow—it's like— oh, there was this one particular one where I was just stopped by two horrible people, and I knew I was going to get it from one of them—it was one of those fatalistic things—and I feel like it's maybe because I have something inside that's terribly valuable—but it's as though I can't really protect myself in a way. And I can't talk to my husband about it. When I have nightmares I never call out when I'm asleep —I just suffer in silence and don't say anything.
>
> CATHERINE: Well, my husband notices mine because I wake up talking, and I'll be just wringing wet, and I hardly ever sweat.

For Mary, the sense of carrying something "terribly valuable" triggered her anxiety. She seemed unsurprised at the positive element, the sense that her baby was so valuable, but was reluctant to tell her husband about the fear, as though there were something wrong with feeling terror during pregnancy.

Women are justifiably concerned about whether or not such extreme and disruptive feelings are normal. They continually need reassurance from each other and from people close to them that they are not the only ones who have been distressed by dreams and fantasies during pregnancy. In the discussion group, the women shared nightmares just as they shared pleasant experiences. Both seemed important and common aspects of their pregnancies.

Often the dreams contained "someone," "those horrible men that come to the door," or threatening animals: "The cat leaped at me and clawed my arm . . . I picked him up and slung him to the wall." Dream symbolism is a shifting and highly personal phenomenon, and there are reservations about making any general interpretations about the meaning of a particular symbol. However, the theme of assault by an "other," malevolent force—another form of the evil eye—is so common that it is worth exploring further. It seems to rise from several important elements of the pregnant state. First, there is a realistic fear by a pregnant woman that if she were to be assaulted or injured in an accident, the consequences would be far greater than usual. Not only she, but also her fetus, is at risk. We have been reminded of this in recent years as caregivers and judges have had to decide whether to terminate the pregnancy of a woman in a coma in order to increase her odds of survival or whether to use her comatose body as an organic incubator until the baby reaches full term.

It is not surprising that women feel increasingly vulnerable to physical assault as their bodies swell and their reactions slow down. The fear of assault may be related to anxiety about the delivery; women may be anxious about losing control of their bodies. Labor contractions are involuntary and, particularly in the first pregnancy, may be seen as alien and separate from a woman's usual functional identity. The doctors and other strangers will, precisely at this most vulnerable time, be probing into the very center of the woman's body. Clearly, her fears of assault are not totally without foundation.

Finally, this fear may be a representation of the woman's own hostility toward the stranger that is increasingly forcing itself into her world. Having entered the uterus, the baby shall one day force itself into her house too. This stranger is probably the symbol that is hardest for a woman to associate with the child, because positive feelings may consciously dominate her experience. Nevertheless, there may be latent and unconscious feelings of fear and resentment and even murderous anger that may be expressed repetitively in such dreams.

Sometimes, women can see the hostility veiled in an unpleasant dream. For example, one three-months-pregnant woman dreamed about fish. To her, the symbol was obvious. "I knew I was caught," she said. "I was pregnant." Other times, another unconscious comment will reveal hidden meaning in a dream. The woman who dreamed about the cat that she "slung" to the wall talked about her feelings concerning her young infant in identical terms after he was born: "He kept on crying and I couldn't get back to sleep. I got to the point where I thought I would slam him against the wall." A woman with slightly less violent impulses repeatedly dreamed she threw her dog through an open window. Neither of these women was ever abusive or inappropriate with her infant.

The logic of dreams is often obscure. A psychotherapist and his or her dream-oriented client may spend hours on the fascinating task of unraveling the many levels of a single dream. The pressing reality of a frightening dream is not a sign of pathological feelings about the pregnancy or a warning that a woman will be a bad mother. A woman should realize that the very intensity of her fear may be related to her positive feelings, to her sense that she is charged with something extremely valuable. Although there *is* the element of fear at her own destructive impulses, it is better to face this aspect of the mother-child relationship during the pregnancy than to experience it as a distorted feeling after the baby actually arrives. We are bound to be ambivalent about anything that disrupts our lives and requires so much selfless attention as an infant.

Many pregnancy dreams contain highly positive themes: ecstatic anticipation, joy at the fullness of life, the love of a man, unity with a world alive with growing things. There are dreams in which the woman is already a mother playing joyously with a grown child. But it is the frightening dreams that are most likely to come up in the presence of a doctor or therapist and especially with other pregnant women. These are the dreams that demand reassurance; these are the dreams that harass the woman who does not realize that the themes they represent are a normal part of pregnancy.

The fear of being trapped also commonly finds expression in the dreams of a pregnant woman, who may be identifying with the baby or experiencing concern about how the door will be unlocked and how the baby will get out. She may also be trapped by the looming responsibilities of motherhood or fear of confinement, particularly in the hospital: "I was locked in the library basement by the director. I was brought bread and water. I was a prisoner for two days and then let out."

A colleague reports a dream that uses fish and water symbolism to express anxiety about assault and the fear of being trapped:

> I was swimming down a muddy river through black reeds and somebody was after me, maybe more than one person. I kept swimming, finally reaching a swimming pool. There were waterfalls or reeds on both sides and I couldn't get by. I woke.[17]

What does this dream mean? Is it total identification with the fetus, even a conception dream of the ovary being chased by sperm and finally reaching the uterus? Or is it a dream about the woman's own experience in pregnancy, of feeling trapped, of being afraid of the world, the people around her, and the emerging person inside? This dream occurred when the woman was only three months pregnant, which may explain some of the confusion between the dreamer and the baby. The fetus had not yet moved, was not yet visible. The woman was only just beginning, painfully, it appears, to achieve some psychological separation from the hardly developed creature lurking inside her. One might view this as a dream in which the dreamer experiences herself both as the pregnant woman and as the helpless fetus.

Dreams about the arrival of the baby are particularly common and usually quite upsetting. For women in their first pregnancy, there is most obviously a concern about their untested competence as mothers. A woman in our discussion group described the classic state:

> I'd dream that I'd had the baby and had forgotten it. For two or three days it had been lying in the bassinet and I hadn't fed it or anything. And it was an all-shriveled thing and it was dying!

Her fear of neglecting the baby is fairly common. Some women dream of losing the baby after it is born; one woman found it, "wrinkled like a dried prune," on the top of a closet.

The fear of "losing" the baby can be much more than simply the woman's anxiety that she will not be a good mother or her feelings of having been neglected when she herself was a baby. It is a dream about what will actually happen—the baby will be "lost" from her uterus. Early in pregnancy, most women worry about having a miscarriage. Later in pregnancy they may be sure they will "lose" the child through delivery. Will it still be theirs? Will they still be able to feed it, protect it, keep it safe and warm? Won't they themselves suddenly be empty, deflated? Psychoanalysts suspect that some postpartum depressions may be related to this sense of loss at the physical separation of the baby from the mother's body. While they may be exaggerating a single aspect of a complex event, they are right to stress the importance of the "death" that occurs along with the birth, for the arrival of an infant entails the loss of a fetus.

Labor contractions and the act of giving birth are often bypassed in dreams. The newborn or, frequently, an older child simply appears. In other dreams the arrival may be somewhat bizarre. It may literally be "delivered" by United Parcel Service. One woman dreamed she was standing on the street corner while her husband picked up the baby. Another dreamed that her baby just emerged one day while she was reclining on the couch. It jumped up next to her, looked in her eyes, then changed into a dog and leaped out the window. A more frightening dream has a similar theme: "The baby was born with only the head. The body was a stick, but this was considered normal."[18] Here is a dream from a woman in her seventh month:

> I dreamed the baby had been born. I don't remember if it was a boy or a girl. I was in the hospital in labor. I felt it was like work. I heard myself thinking, "It is coming." All of a sudden it was there. I thought, "Well, the baby is here! I'd better get up and take care of it." Then I awoke.

It is common, however, for women to dream of bypassing the fragile and barely human infant by having a beautiful, well-developed six-month-old child. "I dreamed once about the baby, a brown-haired, blue-eyed boy of about fifteen pounds." It is no accident that the most common new-baby advertisements depict a well-nourished toddler. Women may know better, but the older child is the one that triggers the least ambivalent response.

Dreams about a child of one particular sex may reflect a woman's attitudes toward her own sexual identity as well as her desire for a child of one sex or the other. One woman reported dreaming about a young man, but as she drew closer, she saw that he was wearing makeup and was, in fact, a woman. This mother-to-be had consciously wanted a boy, but felt fated to have a girl, noting that her relatively small belly and extreme emotional lability were sure signs that she was carrying a girl. Later in the same pregnancy she dreamed of playing with her niece, which she said meant that she was now reconciled to having a girl and was sure that she would be able to love and enjoy the baby even though it was a girl. These dreams might reflect ambivalence about sexual identity almost as though the dreamer consciously assumed the superiority of men but unconsciously wanted to identify with women.

Our discussion of dreams and fantasies has relied on the particular stage of pregnancy as a critical index in understanding the meaning of a particular symbol or anxiety. For example, we have interpreted the dream about the fish swimming down the river as an *early* dream, reflecting the dreamer's confusion as to the identity of the fetus, which she cannot yet distinguish from herself. Similarly, anxiety about injury, which will simultaneously come to the mother and the fetus, seems more characteristic of the first half of pregnancy. By the seventh month, a woman is more likely to dream about losing the baby, which assumes that the fetus has achieved some separateness even though the separation entails danger.

One patient was able to define three distinct phases in her pregnancy. At first she was obsessed with dreams of harm coming to herself. In the middle of the pregnancy, these dreams were supplanted by disturbing thoughts about her husband being hurt or killed, generally in an automobile accident. At the end of the pregnancy, she was increasingly concerned with injury to the baby and was no longer haunted by the threats to herself or her husband. While her dreams may have been more distinct and more clearly related to her conscious concerns than those of most women, her experience may serve as a useful prototype for the developing concerns of pregnant women. In our analysis of the themes that came up in our original discussion group, we discovered that there is a timetable for the psychological events of pregnancy. Although the "stages" are not clearly marked, there are psychological regularities that tend to follow the biological clock. In the next chapters, we will look at the unfolding story of pregnancy within a woman's psyche.

3

The Stages of Pregnancy

THE PSYCHOLOGICAL REALITY of pregnancy is not coextensive with the physiological events. One may feel psychologically and emotionally pregnant before conception has occurred or, more rarely, one may be psychologically and emotionally unaware of pregnancy until a baby is born. We believe that, under optimal circumstances, mind and body will be in synchrony. However, few lives are optimal. At the end of pregnancy, the body's demands are so intense, the mind is sure to be influenced. At the beginning of pregnancy, there is more room for individual variation.

The psychological timetable of pregnancy will never be as precise as its physical counterpart. We cannot know when—or whether—each woman is thinking about her relationship to her mother, worrying about labor, or obsessing about her weight the way we know when the fetal heart begins to beat or when the cervix is ripe. We cannot measure the strength of a woman's trust for her husband or discover her rejection of the baby the way we can measure blood pressure or detect edema. There is much to be learned about the pregnancy experience by studying, stage by stage, the progression of certain themes and concerns through the months.

In spite of the wide range of variation in individual experience and the indefinite nature of psychological issues, we are dividing the pregnancy into the traditional three-month periods called trimesters. In recent years, with the advent of early pregnancy testing and sonograms which can track the development of the fetus, pregnancy is more often timed by weeks rather than trimesters, particularly in the rapid sequence of the first three months, when the fertilized ovum becomes the developing embryo which evolves into the fetus.

As any woman who has waited for the results of chorionic villus sampling or an amniocentesis will know, a week or even a day may seem to make a huge difference in her life. Nevertheless, psychological issues are not as precise as the physiological developments; we retain trimesters as our unit of measurement.

THE FIRST TRIMESTER

Conception

In the past twenty years, the early weeks of pregnancy have changed much more than any other part of the experience. The combined influences of the sexual revolution and women's liberation have created parents who are sophisticated about contraception and more likely to be in control of their fertility. Many women plan ahead to such a degree that they change their diet, take prenatal vitamins, and begin to exercise months before they stop using contraceptives. They are doing everything they can to assure a healthy pregnancy and a healthy baby.

Many couples find that the freedom to make love without contraception adds an extra thrill to their sexual lives. From the woman's experience, sexual intercourse is the beginning of the physical process of being pregnant and giving birth as well as nurturing an infant. Most obviously, it involves the same body parts and same hormonal changes. Sexual arousal is like a mini-childbirth experience complete with gradual arousal, contractions of the reproductive organs, and changes in breasts and external genitalia. Intercourse also entails a process of opening, both emotionally and physically, the woman welcoming the man inside of her body, his sperm swimming up past the cervix, and if fertilization and implantation take place, the baby-to-be settling in the uterus. The woman now must welcome the embryo into her body, open to its presence as it develops into a fetus within her. At the birth she must stretch open even farther, beyond any level she could have imagined possible. The physical accommodation, stretching and opening, seems to have a parallel in a woman's emotional life as she enters the vulnerable condition of pregnancy.

Fertility problems[1]

Technically, infertility means the failure to conceive after a full year of sexual intercourse without contraception. In real life, however, a couple can feel that they have a serious problem well before the end of a year. Failure to conceive even after a month or two can be a disappointment and may lead to concerns about personal and sexual inadequacy. When conception fails month after month, it injures self-esteem and has an unfortunate effect on romance. Sex becomes a scheduled responsibility regulated by the doctor, surrounded by basal thermometer, charts, and everything from weird positions to amulets and vitamin pills.

When conception does not occur, modern medicine may be able to help. Unfortunately, the quest for pregnancy may become virtually an addiction, for there is always the hope that the next month will be different, that the next procedure will be the winner. Most vulnerable to this stress are women near the end of their childbearing years who have postponed childbearing, perhaps even had abortions for unwanted pregnancies, and finally are in a position to welcome a baby. They may become almost frenzied and find themselves obsessed, having difficulty concentrating at work and overcome with anger and resentment when they see women with children. The sight of a pregnant woman can cause them to redden or to burst into tears. They feel that the situation simply isn't fair, and of course it isn't. Women, and especially teenagers, who do not want a baby and don't have the resources to care for it, often conceive when trying not to, and these women who are trying so hard to become pregnant cannot.

After a long period of fear of infertility, pregnancy will be viewed as an especially precious thing. However, the inevitable negative feelings that normally occur during the first trimester may, in this case, be totally unacceptable or may produce undue anxiety. For example, one thirty-two-year-old woman asked for an abortion in her third month of pregnancy. The clinic interviewed her before acting on her request and discovered that she had been a patient at an infertility clinic for a period of five years. In further counseling, she described a flood of negative feelings that did not fit her image of her conscious wishes for motherhood. She had decided that she was unfit to have a baby. With a little reassurance, her anxiety decreased and she realized that her ambivalence was normal, not evidence that she was a bad person. She went on to have a much-wanted baby.

Confirmation and acceptance of pregnancy

A woman no longer has to rely on the old evidence of a missed period or two to find out whether she is pregnant; easy early home pregnancy tests give reliable evidence to confirm a woman's intuition that she has conceived. She can then go to the doctor to have it confirmed.

Once a pregnancy is confirmed and accepted, whether to keep it may become the next issue. The most important task of the first trimester is for the pregnant woman and her partner to accept the reality of their conception and for the woman to come to grips with all that this implies.

The fetus cannot survive outside the womb at this stage of development, just weeks after fertilization. One might even ask the question, when does the fertilized ovum, sometimes called the "product of conception," become a fetus, an individual, an actual child-to-be? Geneticist Clifford Grobstein believes that for the first two weeks after fertilization, before implantation,

> there is no embryo, and the future of the cells that will become an embryo is not fixed. Any one of them, if separated from the others, could conceivably produce a total individual. That's why I think it's important and proper to call this early stage a pre-embryo.[2]

Grobstein says that pregnancy does not begin until implantation, which initiates hormonal changes in the woman. Such a fine distinction in the very early weeks is relevant to people who are conscious of conception and waiting eagerly to find out whether or not they have begun the process of making a baby. It is obviously irrelevant to someone who does not know about the pregnancy until several weeks or months have passed.

At first, it is the pregnancy itself that must be made sure of, revalidated over and over again. Skipped periods, morning sickness, emotional lability, and fatigue can give reassurance (welcome or unwelcome) that the pregnancy is real. Disbelief in the pregnancy is not necessarily a problem early in pregnancy. If a woman is in reasonable health and does not use drugs, cigarettes, or alcohol dangerously, she can wait for the proof of the kicking fetus to convince her that she is indeed pregnant. But denial is often based on fear, and when a woman denies having any fears, she may be expressing an internal conflict and creating more anxiety rather than taking steps to reduce it. Women who want a baby but are afraid of miscarriage are understandably reluctant to invest emotion in the pregnancy and have trouble believing they are genuinely going to have a baby until the second trimester.

Under optimal circumstances, the first trimester is a time of joy, when the secret of the womb is hidden deep within the woman, when she can selectively share it with those whom she chooses to tell. It is hers, it is a change within her body. She can walk down the street and see *really* pregnant women, those already in maternity clothes, and know what they do not know, that she is one of *them*. If she has a bit of nausea, or is more tired than usual, she can smile at it as a happy reminder of what she is doing, of the important work that is going on within her. There is little else to be done. True, for a woman in her first pregnancy, this may be somewhat frustrating. There is no sudden, miraculous change, no need to buy maternity clothes or baby things, hardly even a need to see the doctor. She may change her diet and try to get more sleep—and even these things may be seen as a search for *something* to do.

Deciding whom to tell may take on a gamelike quality. Some women will drop hints from their first missed period. Others hide the information even from their partners until changes become so obvious that the situation must be explained. Still others act as though they do not believe what is happening and do not accept the fact of the pregnancy.

Prenatal testing[3]

We are learning how to diagnose many congenital illnesses from samples of fetal tissue taken from the woman's uterus during pregnancy (in chorionic villus sampling or amniocentesis) or from looking at the image of the fetus on a sonogram screen. New procedures which are less intrusive to the pregnant woman and less dangerous to the fetus are being developed. They can provide accurate results earlier and earlier in the pregnancy. Just a few years ago, amniocentesis results were not available until late in the second trimester. The hope is that a simple blood sample will provide enough information for an accurate reading of fetal chromosomes so that treatment or abortion can be initiated early in the first trimester. The old procedures were emotionally distressing even when the results were happy.

Childbirth educators with whom we have spoken almost always say that a sonogram (a procedure in which an image of the fetus is re-created on a computer screen) is a positive experience for their students and that it facilitates maternal-fetal attachment and paternal-fetal attachment. Women who cannot conceptualize what is happening within them become believers when they see the fetus moving on the screen. We have known women who carried photos of their babies taken from the sonogram screen in their wallets. One in particular, whom we will call Barbara, relied on technology to help her through the entire experience. She was thirty-nine years old when, after years of trying, she finally conceived. Her own mother was an intensely fearful person who had lost a baby at birth and who intensified rather than reduced her daughter's anxiety. Barbara's obstetrician ordered a sonogram every few months, so she had a reassuring peek at her developing baby at regular intervals. The technicians took a Polaroid photograph of the sonogram screen, so Barbara had snapshots of her baby before it was born. She carried this proof that everything was fine with her at all times. Barbara did not have to resort to denial to overcome her fears. She was able to incorporate the baby and see that she was pregnant from the early months.

Not every woman has Barbara's overwhelmingly positive

experience with sonograms. Technological care may seem intrusive rather than supportive. We heard a story of a patient who did not understand English very well. She was so confused by the explanations of the images on the screen that she believed she was carrying a strange assembly of limb fragments that would never come together as a real baby. The procedure was stressful rather than reassuring.

In pregnancy, even more than in other situations that interact with medicine and technology, caregivers must be extremely careful to pay attention to the meaning of the experience to the patient. Because pregnancy and birth are normal biological events that require the active participation of the expectant mother, the "patient" does not benefit from taking on a "sick" role. She benefits from every possible indication that she is a healthy woman carrying a normal fetus and that her body is able to perform the extraordinary tasks that await her.

Couples may go for prenatal screening for no other reason than to learn the gender of the fetus and some have chosen to abort when the fetus was a girl. We read about a future in which the genetic code will be broken and we will be able to analyze all of the information contained in the chromosomes of the embryo or fetus. Will the baby be blond or dark, curly- or straight-haired, tall or short, smart or slow? Will he or she resemble the mother's family or the father's? Will he or she have Grandfather's nose or Grandmother's eyes?

Do we want to know the answers to these questions early in pregnancy, before the fetus has developed into a viable human being, when there is still time to abort? Some people do seem to want to assert control over life's mysteries; others feel they should accommodate to fate and learn to love what they get rather than strive to create what they want.

The idea of terminating a pregnancy is possible as long as the woman conceptualizes pregnancy as a change in her own body, not the life of another person. Once the fetus is conceptualized as alive and aware, the decision becomes much more difficult.

Fetal movement begins at about six weeks, but it is only reflexive movement. Geneticist Grobstein states that, "from 8 to 20 weeks, the central nervous system is so extremely immature, especially the brain, that there seems no possibility of any awareness."[4] A woman and her partner with strong emotional investment in their child may perceive it as sentient, but this is a projection of their wishes, healthy wishes in a wanted pregnancy; nevertheless, they would have a terrible conflict if considering abortion.

Abortion[5]

Like the technology of fertility, legal abortion has changed the psychology of early pregnancy. The current generation of childbearing women do not necessarily assume that if they are pregnant, they are going to have a baby. Some use abortion almost as a form of birth control. We have known women who chose abortion because they had a bout of flu with a high fever the week after conception and were afraid the fever might have damaged the embryo, which is so vulnerable at its earliest stages of development. Other women who want very much to be mothers also want to have control over *when* they have a baby or which pregnancy to keep. If a particular pregnancy feels suspect in some way, if the partner is not supportive or not present, if the career demands are too intense, if the woman just doesn't "feel ready yet," she may choose abortion.

Miscarriage[6]

Most miscarriages occur during the first trimester. To the uninformed, a miscarriage may seem common and expectable. Only about one out of three fertilized ova develops all the way through to a live birth. Many fail to implant and therefore never activate a pregnancy. Many more fail to survive the first three months of the pregnancy. For a woman who has one, however, a miscarriage can be difficult and even tragic. Especially for someone who has already conceptualized the product of her womb as a real person, as her beloved child, the miscarriage is equivalent to the loss of a baby.

Miscarriage is often accompanied by grief and, if unacknowledged, by depression and despair. In addition to the loss is the feeling of inadequacy, of something being wrong with one's reproductive organs. This becomes fear and anxiety in subsequent pregnancies. For a woman who has had one miscarriage, the first trimester (and particularly the period in which the first loss occurred) of the next pregnancy can be extremely tense. We knew a couple who could not relax or socialize when the wife became pregnant after a miscarriage—until they learned the results of the amniocentesis. Then the mother-to-be signed up for childbirth classes (early) and the father-to-be handed out cigars, as though the child were already born!

A woman who has had one or more miscarriages may, consciously or unconsciously, feel that she can only create dead or bad or blighted things. This belief may pervade her sense of herself in all areas and may become projected onto any baby that she does ultimately carry to term. A mother with such a background may startle her family by becoming depressed, rigid, rejecting, guilty, and afraid to attach to a baby that she has been trying so desperately to have for so many years. She needs help appreciating her unconscious fears.

Ambivalence

Ambivalence is normal in the first trimester. When the woman realizes that something might go wrong, that the baby *might* be lost, there may be a certain appeal in this idea, even though she knows it would mean physical and emotional discomfort. There may be an awareness that the discomfort of abortion or miscarriage is far less than the stress of a term pregnancy and child-rearing. If the pregnancy occurred accidentally, the choice to keep the baby is made in this trimester. The "unplanned" baby is often a euphemism. The true meaning behind the apparently random act may range from "trapping" the man into marriage to the unconscious need to be exposed in sexual guilt. Often the decision to keep a pregnancy indicates that, though not consciously planned, the family was ready for a baby.

Physical symptoms

When physical symptoms occur in the first trimester, they may be the first hint a woman has about how unpredictable childbearing can be. There may be weakness, nausea, morning sickness, and even severe vomiting; this may lead a woman to restrict her usual activities, which in turn may make her resent the pregnancy and the baby. Memories of a difficult previous pregnancy or a bad birth experience can add to the tension.

The symptoms of the first trimester may come as a shock to a woman who did not expect her daily life, and particularly her professional life, to be affected until the time of the baby's arrival. Or she may feel well, but be frightened and anxious because of a bad experience with a previous pregnancy or delivery. Second pregnancies are often less romantic and more uncomfortable than the first. She may experience sudden panic about the new or additional responsibilities. She may wonder whether she will be able to go through with it at all. Will she be able to be a mother? Will she be able to handle yet another child? Can they afford a baby?

Virtually everyone experiences first-trimester fatigue to one degree or another. Often, a woman feels only a slight lazy sensation and hopes for an extra hour of sleep. Sometimes, however, a woman is surprised to discover that she barely has the energy to concentrate at work. Since her pregnancy is not yet visible and may not even be confirmed, the symptom is annoying and distressing. She may not know that it is pregnancy related or, worse, she may not realize that it will pass, that her energy will return later in the pregnancy.

As most people know, "morning sickness" can occur any time of day and for some women persists all day and all night, too. At its most benign, it is the slightest revulsion or queasiness at certain odors (typically coffee and tobacco). At its most extreme, it is persistent vomiting that requires medical treatment. Many women throw up once or twice. A few find themselves continuously nauseous, unable to eat and unable to go about their normal lives. For them, early pregnancy may actually be disabling. This situation is more than discouraging; it is a horrible burden that inevitably makes a woman wish she had never become pregnant. Every woman is ambivalent some of the time. A woman who is continually sick will certainly resent the situation.

Most cases of nausea and vomiting clear up by midpregnancy, though not necessarily at the end of the first trimester; Mother Nature does not care about these arbitrary time measures. Difficult cases can go well into the second trimester and a rare case may persist throughout the pregnancy. All cases are cured by time, even if it takes the birth of the child to alleviate the condition.

Four days after her baby was born, Rachel described to us her experience with hyperemesis gravidarum (persistent vomiting) that had been so severe she had to be hospitalized twice during her pregnancy:

> I told my doctor about reading your book and he said, "I hope it didn't make you think your problem is psychological. It is not. It is all hormonal." But I know he is wrong. They

told me to take little sips of water to keep me from dehy-drating, but I would gag on it and throw it back up. I didn't want *anything* to come inside of me and stay there. In your first edition you said that you think hyperemesis gravida may be related to the psychology of anorexia. Now that you are revising it, I hope you say more about that.

Even if hormonal changes trigger the physiological re-sponse, the meaning comes from inside the woman. For Rachel, the meaning was related to intrusion. Secretly, inside herself, she felt that her vomiting during pregnancy meant the same thing to her as her anorexia during ado-lescence. A meaning as important as this needs to be em-braced and understood, not avoided.

At the very least, a woman who is vomiting needs to be soothed and loved and helped to relax so that her body can absorb and hold on to as much food and drink as possible. She needs help taking care of herself so that she can take care of the baby. Persistent vomiting is a situation that can benefit from psychological counseling because the conflicts and feelings evoked by the situation need to be sorted out.

Feelings about work

Women's concerns about working or about their career are a major theme throughout pregnancy. When the subject comes up in the first trimester, it is likely to be expressed as a question: "Will I feel well enough to return to work after the baby is born?" Dedicated career women have no question that they will go back. They are committed to hiring the help they need. The baby will become an extra responsibility, an extra domestic involvement, but will not stop their professional progress. Others are not so confident. They aren't sure they will want to leave the baby, yet they are afraid to give up a good job. Marriage is no longer any guarantee of security.

Modern women go into pregnancy knowing that they have a better than 50 percent chance of becoming single mothers before their children grow up. A job is more than a way to earn self-esteem or to have outside stimulation. It is a necessary part of economic security. Couples that have been living for years in a two-paycheck household will suffer a major setback if the new mother does not go back to work. The new father may have to take on a second job. Early in the pregnancy, these issues are frightening, but abstract. Actual planning is just beginning. The fatigue and nausea so common in the first trimester may bring the first realistic glimpse of the problems entailed in trying to "have it all."

Body image

The first trimester is a time when there may be strange fantasies and dreams about the unknown, unseen, and unfelt organism growing inside a woman's body. She may have noticed that even though she has not gained a significant amount of weight, she cannot button her skirts and that her blouses and bras are getting uncomfortable. Her muscles have started to stretch in preparation for the changes that are going to occur later. Her breasts may already have swollen to the full size they will reach. Although her figure has changed ever so slightly, a woman may view these changes as huge. She may feel fat and ugly, or she may be proud of her newly enlarged breasts. But during the first trimester the pregnant woman is probably thinking of what is happening to *her*, for the baby has not yet demanded much attention as a separate being.

Some women remove themselves as far as possible from their biologically determined selves. For them, the physical side of pregnancy may seem alien, uncomfortable, and unwelcome. They may feel they have little need to experience the stages of pregnancy and the progression from conception through birth. They would prefer to parent from a clearly separated position, more like a traditional father. The pregnancy is irrelevant to such a woman's personal sense of her self. Nevertheless, if she does create a baby in the traditional way by carrying the fetus in her uterus rather than adopting, she will have the same bodily changes and feel the baby kick within. But she is less likely to become engaged in the process or to experience many of the psychological changes we are describing in this book.

Sexuality[7]

During the first trimester, sexual appetites vary greatly. Physiological changes may account for these reactions. Breast tissue has enlarged and the added swelling that occurs with sexual arousal is sometimes uncomfortable or even painful. Fatigue and nausea sap a woman's energy and reduce her interest in making love or even in displaying affection. Psychological and social factors seem to be much more important. Masters and Johnson reported an overall decrease in sexual tension and sexual performance during the first trimester in primiparous women, with little change in multiparous women.[8] Many men and women are afraid that sexual activity will injure the fetus. They may have trouble expressing this fear to their partners, but it inhibits spontaneous contact between them. If the pregnancy is a time of great upheaval or insecurity, sexual concerns are overwhelmed by other personal worries.

Those who feel that sex is intended primarily for childbearing may have scruples about indulging in sex after conception has taken place. For some, their new potential role of mothering changes the meaning of sexual pleasure and provokes guilt and remorse. They may become hypersensitive, afraid to be touched, repulsed at their enlarged breasts, and unwilling to be reminded of their sexuality. However, many others feel an increased sexual desire. Some report reaching orgasm too fast and feeling so erotic that they are afraid of frightening their husbands; others become obsessed with thoughts of ingesting the semen to help the baby grow. Still others experience a more indolent sensuality and want to be pampered and played with, to be taken care of and kept secure.

The changes in sexual feelings and the sudden mood swings of pregnancy may reinforce one another and upset even the most stable marital situation. One woman described her own confusion at breaking out into tears at the end of a particularly ecstatic orgasm. Her husband was mystified and hesitant to initiate sex again. Almost every couple must work more intimately together to cope with their shifting sexuality and emotionality. The relationship has acquired a new meaning even if the pregnancy has not forced physiological changes upon the sexual response pattern.

Interest in other mothers

As a woman realizes she is actually going to become a mother, she becomes intently concerned with her own mother, her mother-in-law, and other women who have been maternal figures in her life. She may begin to worry about what kind of mother she will be and how she will relate to her children's grandmothers. "How can I help being like my mother if she is the only model I have?" a woman may ask. She may want desperately to do better than her mother has done, but in identifying with her she may feel bound to repeat her mother's mistakes. This conflict was evident in Mary, an independent woman who had moved to a city far from her parents and had had little contact with her mother in years. Suddenly, she started dreaming of her mother, talking with her mother, worrying about her mother. Will she be the "wicked witch" who comes and takes the baby away, because, after all, she is the "real" mother? Another woman remarked, "My mother-in-law didn't have any daughters and this is her first grandchild. I almost feel it won't be my child if it is a girl. I hope it is a boy." For other women there is the possibility that their own mothers will be the good fairies who will protect and guide the daughter and infant. For most, there are simply questions: Will she approve or disapprove? Who will be the boss when both are mothers? How will she act? How will she react when her advice is ignored?

Occasionally we see a woman whose mother remains the most important figure throughout pregnancy. The daughter may, in fact, be having the baby for her mother, either to replace a child the mother has lost or to compensate for the mother's inability to have a baby anymore. This is most likely to occur with young women who are living with their parents and who know their mothers will assume major responsibility for the baby. There are also subcultures in rural areas and in certain minority groups in which the grandmother is expected to take the major role in child-rearing while the mother leads a relatively separate life.

While women do not truly resolve the problem of their changed relationship to their own mothers until well after the baby is born, the preoccupation with their mothers seems gradually to fade once the second trimester of pregnancy has begun.

THE SECOND TRIMESTER

Months four through six, the second trimester, are called the quiet months. The threat of miscarriage is generally over. Morning sickness, if it occurred, has usually passed. If the woman resisted the idea that she was pregnant, she has probably started to believe and accept the reality. On some days she may find herself shopping for maternity clothes before she absolutely needs them, on others she might still be rummaging through racks of dresses of her nonpregnant size. The initial joy at discovering she was pregnant may have given way to thoughts about the consequences and problems of actually becoming a mother. She may be shopping for baby furniture or redecorating a room for the baby in order to get something concrete and external that she can use to deal with her feelings about the baby. One woman said, "I was able to *look* at cribs this week, but still can't get myself to buy one." Another bought a stroller early in the second trimester and kept it set up in her living room. At the other extreme, a lonely woman waited until her ninth month to begin looking for an apartment that would be adequate for the new family, leaving her still anxious about a new home when labor began.

Examining a woman's response to maternity clothes and baby supplies can reveal much about her feelings and interests for her pregnancy and her coming child. If she does not yet feel attached, she still has time. Working women with demanding jobs are particularly likely to postpone their shopping until the final weeks of pregnancy.

Prenatal bonding

It takes a leap of faith to connect the physical symptoms of pregnancy with the little baby who won't be in the world for another six months. Several specific events change the mother's ability to believe in the fetus. They include hearing the fetal heartbeat in the doctor's office; viewing the fetus on a sonogram screen; receiving positive test results (if there was reason to suspect a problem); and, universally, quickening, the experience of the fetus moving in the womb.

The most overwhelming experience of the second trimester is feeling the baby move. Even if a woman was able to accept the reality of her pregnancy in her first trimester, the proof of it will come in the second. She may become silent and introspective, listening for every gas bubble and interpreting it as movement, almost afraid to hope that the fluttery feeling is really a separate life within her. A sudden secret smile can light her face as, unknown to the rest of the world, a slippery, fishy motion occurs in her womb. Women seem to delight in talking about the sensations of quickening at this stage of pregnancy. The word *quick* means alive, an archaic and charming word that implies the separation of the living from the nonliving at both ends of the life cycle.

Women try to guess whether their baby is a boy or a girl by the way it turns or bumps, ripples or twitches. Generally, the reaction is romantic: "There! Again! Soft as the brush of a butterfly's wing, fragile as a dewdrop trembling on a leaf, she felt her baby move."[9] The discomforts and complaints that may accompany descriptions of movement in the last trimester are seldom present here. Even women who are angry about the discomforts of pregnancy may find relief in feeling the movement. "It means that I don't just have a deformed body, but it's really doing something now." If a woman has feared miscarriage, she may now be sure that the baby is alive and well.

A few years ago, when amniocentesis results did not get back until well into the fifth month of pregnancy, some women who were afraid that they might have to abort the fetus did not feel fetal movement until they received the good news that they had a viable fetus and could carry the pregnancy to term. In other words, they were emotionally unable to feel what was going on inside their wombs because they could not acknowledge the reality of the baby.[10]

Movement is usually perceived between the eighteenth

and twenty-first weeks of pregnancy. This is the time in an old-fashioned pregnancy when the fetus begins to assert its presence. Women who have had sonograms may have seen the fetus move, but now the internal sensations may be associated with a baby they have seen on the screen, and the baby is even more of a reality in their life. As the baby gives dramatic evidence of being present, the pregnant woman starts to conceptualize it as an individual, separate from herself. The changes are no longer just in herself; suddenly there are changes in the *fetus*.

In a high-tech pregnancy, the parents may already know their baby's gender. Some reports suggest that this knowledge begins to shape the parents' relationship to the child. They use different words to describe the movement of a fetus they know to be male than they do to describe a fetus they know to be female.[11] The fetus is being given an identity.

In group meetings, the women were uncharacteristically positive when they compared the various sensations of movement. When asked about negative aspects of the movement, there was a silence. Finally, one member tried very hard to come up with something negative. "All that moving and kicking was starting to make me feel like the pregnancy should get over so that the little guy could shift for himself," she said. But this "negative" comment seemed, rather, to demonstrate a healthy acceptance both of the pregnancy and the reality of the coming baby. The rest of the women apparently agreed, for the remark was greeted with laughter. Late in the pregnancy, the fetal movements are often felt as intrusive and irritating. At this stage, they are a pleasant confirmation that the pregnancy is happening for a reason.

Pregnancy is a time when the mother can hold on to her fantasies about her baby and about herself as a mother while still preparing for the reality. Ruth learned that she was pregnant with a second boy. She had wanted a girl very badly. For two months, she grieved the loss of the little girl of her fantasies. She dreamed of being with a little girl, then she dreamed of being the only woman in an all-male group, and, finally, in the middle of the second trimester, she dreamed she was walking across the street with a little girl and all of a sudden the child disappeared. Ruth realized that she had let go of her expectation for a daughter from this pregnancy and felt herself eager for the birth of her second son. She used pregnancy as a chance to bond to the child she was actually going to have.

Body image

As the baby begins to kick and prove its individuality for the first time, several interesting phenomena may occur. A woman may put on a great deal of weight, trying to enlarge her size so that there will be no question in the eyes of the world that she is truly pregnant. Now that *she* is more sure of it, she may want everyone *else* to know it too, and be frustrated that, in fact, only those who know her well can detect the change and guess its cause. Other women, who have gained a great deal of weight early in the pregnancy as though to convince themselves that it is real, may be able to control their eating now that they have internal proof of the pregnancy.

A woman who gains little or no weight is making a very clear statement about her need to maintain a stable sense of her body image. Her concern for her appearance needs to take into account her own and her baby's nutritional requirements.

In traditional Japanese families, women are presented with an abdominal binder in a small ceremony during the fifth month of pregnancy. When she wraps her *hara obi* around her body, a woman acknowledges her condition. As in all aspects of pregnancy, a woman may respond to this with delight or abhorrence:

> One young mother described the donning of the abdominal sash as a mystical experience that heightened her awareness of her pregnant state. Another young mother, less enthusiastic, complained that the custom was old-fashioned and uncomfortable, but explained that her mother and doctor had talked her into wearing it. [12]

The ceremonial act became a focus for the pregnant woman's feelings about her body and the pregnancy.

Most women will be concerned about whether the particular way in which their bodies are growing or their babies are kicking is in fact normal. They may start to be afraid of their changing bodies or afraid of injuring the baby, now that it has a life of its own. Can they sleep on their stomachs? Is it normal for the belly button to pop out that way? Does the baby kick you in the groin? At mid-pregnancy, the body image has changed so much that a woman must question what is normal.

It will now be clear that the baby is going to force its changes on the woman. She may realize for the first time that she *cannot* control these changes, for they are being caused by the strange creature inside of her. If she tries to gain or lose weight, she will still not be able to modify her silhouette as radically as the baby will. Dreams about injury to the self start to be replaced by dreams about something happening to somebody else, or by dreams about a stranger. A woman may become frightened for the first time.

Dependency needs

With a woman's fear that she cannot control the changes of pregnancy comes the question: Who will now take care of me? Then the concern about her own mother enters a new phase. In the first trimester, the interest was likely to be about motives for becoming pregnant and curiosity about what kind of mother she would be. Now it is more likely to be a desperate search for the figure who has always taken care of her. It seems natural to turn to her mother because, after all, she has borne children, she has experienced pregnancy, she will know what it is like in a way no one else can understand. This is a strongly regressive pull. In most cases a more adaptive solution is to turn away from the past and toward the family of the future.

A woman may shift her dependency from her mother to her partner. She may express frustration that he cannot yet feel the stirring of the baby. She wants him to know that he is already a father, that he is involved in the pregnancy even if he does not carry the baby. It is suddenly important that the partner be able to participate, that he take an interest, that he become a figure upon whom the woman can depend.

A pregnant woman seems to complain to her partner to see whether or not he is concerned. If he responds with a superficial "everything is going to be fine," she may get irrationally angry. "That makes me want to escalate my feelings," Susan told us. "I think the baby is going to be all right and that we'll all survive, but that doesn't mean *everything* will be *fine*. He just doesn't want to listen to the details or know what I'm experiencing."

One study of women who were having their first babies noted that women seemed to express anger at their husbands from the twenty-first to the twenty-fourth week in the pregnancy.[13] The high divorce rate forces a woman to wonder whether her partner will be with her through her child-rearing years. Friendship with other women may, for some, be more important than the less secure trust in the marital relationship. Pregnancy support groups and childbirth preparation classes not only provide information, they also bring a pregnant woman into contact with other women in the same situation. Many intimate relationships grow from the shared experience of pregnancy and early child-rearing.

Part of the psychological importance of needing to be close to the husband rather than a female figure at this stage is probably rooted in contemporary culture. The husband's presence is critical in our mobile society, where the grand-mother is often not around to help take care of her pregnant daughter or help with a new baby. As we shall see in the chapter on the expectant father, it is now often the husband who will have to take charge when the pregnant woman cannot. He may have the important task of reassuring the woman that she is still beautiful and sexy to him, that he can cope with getting his own meals when she is unable to do so, that he can help her with the care of the infant in the early months. Perhaps, too, as the baby moves, it re-minds the woman that the creature within is *his* and *theirs* as much as it is *hers*.

Sexuality

Women often feel more erotic in the second trimester. Much of the physical discomfort, the nausea, fatigue, and insomnia have disappeared. There is less ambivalence about the pregnancy, yet the physical changes are still unremark-able, particularly in the primipara. This increased sexuality expresses itself in interest in sexual encounters and in sexual fantasies and dreams. In the Masters and Johnson studies, 80 percent of the women described a significant improve-ment in sexual relations during the second trimester. Some had satisfactory sexual experiences for the first time in their marriages.[14]

There are some physiological changes that help account for these shifts. Vaginal lubrication is greater at this time.

Also there is increased blood flow to the pelvic area as a function of the enlarging uterus and its contents. This means, first, that the engorgement of the erotic areas probably occurs more rapidly and, secondly, the excitation may continue after orgasm because of the slowness with which these areas return to a near-normal state. Some women complain that, although they are easily excitable and have intense climaxes, they continue to feel desire when the warmth of satisfaction should have enveloped them.

Relationship with the partner

A woman's increased sexual needs are probably minor compared to her new emotional involvement with her husband. She may become overly concerned for his safety. In Chapter 2, we described dreams of the husband being killed or injured. These are particularly intense in women whose own father died or left the family around the time of their own birth or the birth of a sibling. There may be some jealousy about having to share the pregnancy with the husband, now that it is clearly visible and after the movements can be felt by him as well as by her. Some women become hypercritical of their husbands' attitudes, their manners, and their masculinity at this time.

Psychoanalysts have described pregnancy as a fulfillment of a woman's penis envy. At last, so it is alleged, after going through life without a visible external sex organ, the woman has a full, fertile, protuberant belly to prove her value to the world. She has something so important that now men should envy her, for she is doing something that they cannot do. Won't he have womb envy? Won't her partner feel inadequate? Won't he be jealous of the baby, who is so much closer to his wife than he can be himself? This concern over the husband's jealousy and the curiosity about his feelings of adequacy parallel the pregnant woman's attitudes toward her mother. It seems as though the pregnant woman, especially in her first pregnancy, moves from concern about competition with and dependency upon her mother into concern about competition with and dependency upon her husband. This progression, of course, takes on individual patterns in each family. For a woman having a baby in a traditional family, working out the shift in dependency from that of daughter to that of wife is the major psychological task of the second trimester.

Obviously, both mother and husband are of such overwhelming importance that they will be critical at every stage of pregnancy, but in these "quiet months" that potential confusion can be clarified most directly, for while the fact of the pregnancy is firmly established, the child is not yet frighteningly imminent. It is an opportune time for a major reevaluation of the critical relationships in a woman's life.

This is a much larger task for primiparas than multiparas. The multipara has probably already worked out her identity in relationship to her mother and her husband. Her task in the middle period of pregnancy is more likely to be to establish a proper ambience in which to prepare for the slower pace she anticipates for the last months of the pregnancy. She will probably direct her emotional energy into preparing her existent household for the coming change on the assumption that her role in her immediate and in her extended families will remain fairly stable.

THE THIRD TRIMESTER

The third trimester combines pride and fulfillment with anxious anticipation of the imminent unknown and physically uncomfortable event of birth. Now the reality of the pregnancy is inescapable. Most women have resolved their ambivalent attitudes. While in some studies as many as 50 percent of the women in the first trimester openly admitted to not wanting their babies, it is rare for a woman in the third trimester to voice this sentiment. Negative feelings can be easily displaced onto physical discomfort and possible unpleasant expectations of the birth experience. A woman may become aware of the special prerogatives of pregnancy and truly appreciate them for the first time.

In a group of women, a pregnant woman is likely to be dominant, unless there is someone else more pregnant than she, or a mother with a tiny newborn. In the doctor's office, she will feel quite special, and perhaps even conspicuous as the magazine rests on her protruding belly or her blouse bounces around in a most undignified way when the baby kicks. The nurses will know her, for she is coming more frequently and receiving the extra attention of more appointments. Others may get up to give her a chair in a crowded room. Even comparative strangers may pat her on the belly. Neighbors, clerks in the grocery store, as well as her husband, will be solicitous about helping her. She may shrug off the attention as silly or unnecessary—or she may appreciate it as exceedingly helpful. She may very much need to be taken care of, to have help with packages, to sit rather than stand. If she doesn't actually *need* this type of assistance, she may nevertheless feel her status entitles her to certain special privileges. On the other hand, her fear of being helpless may drive her to ignore offers of aid, to deny any need to slow down.

The experience of a biologically based dominance, of identity beyond the personal, of acceptance or deference by formerly indifferent groups of people, can be a very heady affair indeed for some women. Many will feel an almost mystical identification with a primitive feminine principle within them and a closeness with the reproductive, generative elements of the species and, indeed, of all living organisms. The experience is often religious and transcendent.

Feelings about work

The last trimester is a time when the problems of daily life cause the greatest hardships. For primiparas, the last trimester may be annoying and frustrating. Women who feel well, competent, and unaffected by the physical strains of their condition may be happy to continue working until the final week of pregnancy. Others want to take off to prepare their homes for the baby or simply to rest for the final, physically demanding weeks. Women may also want very much to keep busy so that they will not have to think of the frightening unknowns of childbirth.

When they talk of work at this stage in the pregnancy, women are likely to consider the reality of the baby. They are aware of the demands on their body; they aren't sure they will have the energy (or the interest) to return to work. By now, they have fallen in love with their idea of the baby. As a woman in a support group said:

> I hate the idea of returning to work and handing the baby over to someone else—but how would I get ego strokes as a housewife? I don't know anything about taking care of a baby, but it is going to be mine. I just don't know what to do. Maybe a nanny will know more than I do.

Most women assume they will resume work, but they are often unsure how they will combine it with their new role as mother.

Prenatal bonding

Throughout the last three months, women talk continuously about the baby, what it will be like and how they will take care of it, as though the baby is now a real person with its own identity, although it must remain sexless and nameless a little longer for those who have not learned its gender from prenatal testing. There are many joking conversations about what it will look like. Will it have my husband's nose? My chin? Will it be bald? Will its hair fall out later? The endless speculation can go on and on.

After twenty-three weeks, the fetus can survive a premature birth. The baby will be at risk and require intensive care, but it can survive. From this point on, a woman may feel like an especially wonderful, god-created incubator. If she has had signs of premature labor, she may understand that she is the most exquisite environment for her baby.

Naming can become a fascinating topic for a couple who are struggling to individualize the unknown creature. For example, one couple simply could not settle on a name for their first child. They had not thought much about child-rearing as a part of their marriage and had even considered remaining child-free. When the wife actually became pregnant, they were excited and delighted, but had trouble conceiving what it would really be like to have a baby. None of their friends had young children and nothing in their life-style made it easy for them to imagine having children. They did not find a suitable name until after the birth, when they chose a name that seemed to suit the baby they held in their arms. They were more prepared for the second child and settled on two names (one for a boy and one for a girl) in the second trimester, although the choice, again, required a great deal of discussion. When they learned that they were to have a third child, they found two names immediately and kept to them through to delivery. This couple was eager to have each of its children, but had trouble conceptualizing what a baby would actually be like. By the time they were pregnant with the third child, their identity as parents was firmly established, and they felt secure in giving their unborn child an identity of its own. Although naming may be an activity of any trimester, it is primarily in the third trimester that it serves the particularly valuable function of helping a family prepare for a child that will be arriving soon.

Dreams

The dreams of the third trimester are most often about babies, children, and delivery. There may be anxiety dreams about losing or misplacing the baby, or being trapped in a small place and not being able to squeeze out. The dreams reflect reality; in the last months, there are important things to prepare for. The mother-to-be must get ready for labor and childbirth and for the care of the infant itself. All of the work of pregnancy pivots here; a great deal about the adaptation of a couple and their ideas about the future can be assessed by watching their reactions to the acute stress of birth.

Labor and childbirth

Concern and preparation for labor and birth will rival even concerns for the baby during a pregnant woman's final trimester. She has known for nine months that the pregnancy will culminate in childbirth, but now, as her uterus contracts more and more frequently, and her near-term fetus kicks more and more vigorously, she is being constantly reminded that the pregnancy must come to an end, and that there is no easy or magical way for the baby to emerge. Labor may then seem like a journey into the unknown, a journey whose outcome is both uncertain and irrevocable. A woman can hardly avoid concentrating on, even being obsessed by, the way in which her child will get out.

A few women will be forced to take it easy because of the fear of premature labor. If the obstetrician or midwife detects preliminary changes in the cervix or suspects that the uterus is unusually irritable, he or she may prescribe bed rest in the last trimester. Every week in the womb is a great benefit for the fetus, even if it is developed enough to survive outside. Bed rest may be extremely frustrating for a woman used to working and being active. Suddenly she cannot even prepare her own meals or do her laundry. She becomes dependent on her partner's care. Her days may be lonely; boredom may be the hardest work of the pregnancy.

Body image

In the last trimester, a woman's body image is almost discontinuous with her usual physical state. Even for the multipara, the abdomen may seem to swell beyond her previous memories. If she got her body back into shape after the first one, she may be appalled to see it stretch out again, more than before. She is older this time. Will she ever get her figure back?

One primipara said she spent hours in front of the mirror staring at her profile in stark disbelief. At some point, most women will suspect they are carrying twins—how else to account for the bulk and the amount of activity in the uterus? Surely it must be two boys, fighting! Some women smile beatifically at this thought, while others turn pale with fright. Husbands, too, have strong feelings about their wives' new bodies. Some are proud watching their wives move "in her new awkward way," laden with the proof of their masculinity. Others may be repelled by the larger-than-life proportions of swollen breasts and bellies.

Dependency needs

Most women have a pervasive fear in the third trimester: Will there be enough love to go around? Everybody is going to need love: the baby, the husband, the older child, the dog, and the woman herself. Can so much love be found?

For all these reasons, a woman needs extra reassurance in the final weeks of pregnancy. She may turn most intensely to her husband for this. She may wonder if he can still love her when she is so different from the woman he married. She may feel ugly and sloppy and hopelessly removed from the arena of attractive women. Even if a man reassures her that he does love her, he may be unable to demonstrate his feeling sexually.

Sexuality

Heightened sexuality seems to continue into the middle of the third trimester. But here, as in the first trimester, psychological and physical factors may be preeminent and get in the way of sexual expression. The wife's abdomen may present an insurmountable obstacle for a couple whose sexual practices have always been conservative. The best ways to get around the big belly are to use manual stimulation, exotic postures, or oral sex.[15] Unfortunately, some couples who have not experimented with these forms of sexual expression earlier in their relationship feel guilty resorting to them late in pregnancy.

Only rarely do medical concerns prohibit sexual intercourse or orgasms for the pregnant woman late in pregnancy, either because of concern about stimulating early labor or because of fear of infection if the bag of waters, shielding the baby from the outside world, is not intact. More commonly, a couple is too anxious, preoccupied, or uncomfortable to be interested in sex. The fear of hurting the child persists. Awkwardness and reserve about trying new positions are also common.

Sexual tension and frustration can add an unpleasant element to an already anxious phase of pregnancy. Some couples may have abstained since the first trimester, and others may ignore all prohibitions.

The specific solution chosen by a couple is probably less important than their method of reaching their solution. Where communication lapses, a couple finds itself in a sad and lonely situation which may worsen after delivery, when the woman's perineum will be sore and the threat of hemorrhage present, in other words, when another prohibition will be in effect. Lactating breasts and crying infants can do as much to inhibit a man as a huge belly and a kicking fetus. Again, the honesty of shared feelings is the best way to overcome this touchy problem which is common to all couples.

Final preparations

The third trimester is the time to make all the final preparations, unless there will be someone at home to do it all for the mother while she is in the hospital. Most women take comfort and pleasure in getting a layette ready. Handling the clothes gives them a chance to realize the actual size of the newborn, and to visualize its need: diapers, soap, blankets. Each item reflects an aspect of this phenomenon that will be with them soon.

Superstitions about baby items are widespread. Many couples will not bring anything into the house until the baby is born. Marie was afraid of all preparations:

> People keep giving me things and I hide them. I had a friend who had six showers, and then the baby died. I wish nobody would give me anything.

Other women focus on just one or two, such as buying the announcements or addressing the envelopes. Most agree that it is practical to get these tasks done before the baby is born, but they are nervous about it. Philippa was an exception. She was scheduled for a repeat cesarean section and was confident that all would go well. She filled out the announcements in advance, including the baby's name, gender, and date of birth. She knew everything except length and weight!

Physical discomfort

Insomnia is one of the most common complaints of late pregnancy. One woman said that her husband had to sleep on the couch because the baby "kicked him out of bed." The unborn infant was keeping them both up. Another woman waited for her husband to go to sleep and then turned on a light and read each night. Other women find it impossible to sleep without their husbands. Women in the last trimester may have an intense need to hold something or someone. A husband may happily gratify this need. Puppies, kittens, pillows, and stuffed animals serve also, especially during the day. The sight of a tiny infant may virtually make a woman's arms ache for someone that size to hold.

Anger and resentment may resonate in a woman's voice when she describes a near-term fetus pounding away at her vital organs or worries about the baby kicking through her abdominal wall. As the uterus fills up more and more of the abdomen, she worries about the stomach, the diaphragm, or the ribs being pushed out of the way, about the bladder being irritated—which does happen, causing embarrassing accidents and perhaps encouraging her to feel infantile and dependent. Drooling may also occur, and may be very threatening to a woman who is trying hard to prepare herself for motherhood but finds herself acting more like an infant herself, wanting only to curl up in a warm place with a furry toy.

The eighth month may actually be the most uncomfortable time of pregnancy, for then the baby has reached almost its maximum size but has not yet settled down into the pelvis ready to be delivered. A woman may feel that her veins are swollen, her breath hard to catch. She may wonder how she can continue to get larger and have more strain on her organs for yet another month. In fact, she may be far *more* comfortable and have more energy in the ninth month because the baby's head drops deep into the pelvis and relieves pressure on the diaphragm. Unfortunately, many women react to this renewed energy with an intense urge to bustle around and *do* things this last month. They start a redecorating project or try to accomplish everything that they might as easily have taken care of earlier, like the woman who did not look for a new apartment until the ninth month. This spurt of activity may be accelerated by a woman's anxiety about losing control at the birth, by depressing feelings about the possible loss of the baby, and by the added responsibilities she will so soon acquire. If she remains inactive, she may wonder how she will bear the anticipation. How will she keep from thinking that each isolated contraction is the first of the irreversible chain that will lead to the birth of her baby? But if she tries to start a new project, what happens if she gets caught off guard and begins labor with unfinished business at home? Or what if she gets overtired one day and goes into labor that night, before she can catch up on her rest? And so on.

Typical of the final weeks of pregnancy are a general restlessness, insomnia, water retention, and, especially, swollen feet. The baby is often felt as separate and intrusive. Occasionally a woman has a sudden burst of energy, often attached to an intense hope that labor is beginning. By the end, most women are ready to have pregnancy become a thing of the past.

For the multiparas, the last trimester also becomes an

increasingly anxious period. Too many physicians and husbands assume that pregnancy is easy for "old-timers." Presumably they already know what it is all about, already have proven themselves as mothers, and therefore don't need any extensive preparation for childbirth or infant care. They have already worked out a life-style that copes with mothering whether it includes outside work or not. Unfortunately, our experience suggests the opposite. With other young children at home, a pregnant woman cannot trot out to exercise classes, shop for new maternity clothes, search for the perfect cradle. She has the basic equipment, although it may look a bit shoddy to her now. She may be told to take naps, but can't when her four-year-old doesn't. The thrill of a new life within her may be mitigated by the memory of the insistent demands of an earlier infant, who may have "cried and cried all night."

True, there are profound joys to balance the anxieties—comparison of the movements of this fetus with the last, pride at not having gained as much weight, security in knowing that her family will be able to cope with the "newcomer." But the subject of labor and delivery looms larger and larger as the last trimester evolves—and for the multipara, it is *not* an unknown. There may have been a complication that made an earlier delivery particularly difficult. She is older now. She is more likely to have had physical complications related either to pregnancy or to other times in her life. (Fatigue is especially likely to become a factor when a pregnant woman cannot take good care of her health because of the demands of her other children.) She knows that things *can* go wrong. If she has had a cesarean section, she has the difficult choice between more surgery or a VBAC, a vaginal birth after cesarean.

Multiparas are particularly likely to have an uncomfortable sense that the baby may arrive at any moment in the last two months, wherever they are, whatever they are doing.

Preliminary contractions, which may pass unnoticed in a first pregnancy, may be strong enough to urge a woman to call her doctor or even to take a premature trip to the hospital in subsequent pregnancies. A woman may be thrilled at the sudden tightening of her uterus, proud that her body is preparing to play its role. However, frequent sporadic contractions can be wearing on a woman's nerves. Throughout the last month she may be referring to her watch and questioning endlessly whether these contractions are "real" or not. With all of the modern talk about painless childbirth, she may believe that her labor contractions will be no different from these, that delivery may be imminent even though there has been no "show" and the bag of waters has not broken. She is likely to have heard stories about women who had babies unexpectedly at home, or who had to spend six weeks or more in bed to prevent a sensitive uterus from contracting to expel a premature baby. She is far less likely to have been told that many women experience contractions from the sixth month of pregnancy on. Thus she may live through her last month hour by hour, interminably waiting for the tension in her uterus that causes her to catch her breath and breathe more deeply, the contractions that indicate labor is truly established.

Our focus in this chapter has been on the experiential distinctions between each trimester of pregnancy. There are different problems at each stage and each of these engenders anxiety as an inevitable consequence of the rapid changes taking place. Yet it would be a mistake to leave this chapter with the impression that anxiety is the root experience. On the contrary, the overwhelming sense is that of ecstasy. The excitement of carrying an invisible fetus in the first trimester is as intense and romantic as falling in love. It brings on the same spurts of joy, the same desire to sing and skip down the street, the same feeling of being more special than anybody else in the world. If that happiness starts to fade, it is renewed by the baby's first movements, for now the woman has a chance to fall in love with her state all over again.

Finally, in the ninth month, a woman reaches one of the most beatific phases of human existence. She acquires a physical form that has stimulated not only art but worship throughout the ages. Her smile may surpass the Mona Lisa's. Her presence will affect everyone in the room. Friends may pat her tummy in greeting, or ask to sit next to her to enjoy her radiance. She may be teased, but in a loving way, as if everyone were trying to participate vicariously in what she is doing. She may not fit the *Playboy* image of femininity, but she will epitomize another kind of womanly beauty. Men will see her as a full, rich vessel. Some may say that their image of the most beautiful scene in the world is that of a woman eight and a half months pregnant running across an open field. Photographers and painters have captured this state best when they show the pregnant woman standing serenely at a window, emphasizing the extent to which her experiential world is taking place on the inside, but with a reminder that it is on the brink of making the transition, of passing through the window into the world beyond.

4

Birth

THE MEANING OF CHILDBIRTH

CHILDBIRTH, with its personal drama, risk of death, its significance for survival of the family, tribe, race, and even species, is almost universally marked by rituals and ceremonies, only some of which are directly related to the actual task of helping a mother deliver a child. Cultures vary widely in the nature of their observances and practices at childbirth, but almost every society does something special.

The diverse cultural backgrounds of American families complicate the pattern of responses to labor and birth. The choices of behavior in one family may seem bizarre to another's prejudices, but in a sense it is no more peculiar for an expectant father, a witch doctor, and a midwife to simulate labor and confinement in a specially constructed hut while the wife inconspicuously delivers the baby elsewhere than it is for a husband to wait out the birth watching a football game in a local bar while his wife labors in the presence of strangers in an unfamiliar white hospital cubicle.

American women of the past few decades have shared a romantic fantasy about "natural" childbirth, a fantasy that says that "primitive" women give birth easily and with no pain, that the difficulties of childbirth are by-products of the neuroses of civilization. Fortunately, a generation of female anthropologists has studied childbirth in a wide range of "primitive" settings and reports back a more realistic view of the "natural" condition of giving birth. As one of them, Brigitte Jordan, writes in no uncertain terms, " 'primitive childbirth' is neither primitive, nor painless, nor natural."[1] Elsewhere she states:

> There are some women in any society who give birth without experiencing pain . . . [but] pain is a recognized and expected part of the birth process in almost all societies . . . the notion that "primitive" birth is easier than "civilized" birth is clearly false.[2]

The myth that primitive cultures have an easier time in childbirth persists even in the face of evidence of maternal and fetal death rates in primitive cultures. Perhaps the example most often cited is an incident from the Pearl Buck novel *The Good Earth*, in which a Chinese peasant gives birth and then immediately returns to work in the fields. We seem to forget that childbirth is only conducted this way under conditions of extreme poverty and/or degradation and that such circumstances are associated with high infant and maternal death rates.

A wounded soldier does not expect a battle to stop because he is wounded; he may have to endure an amputation without anesthesia. But the same man would surely receive concerned attention for the same injury under other circumstances. Humans heal more easily when they receive loving attention. Folk practices of "laying on of hands" do bring about "miraculous" cures just as appropriate support eases childbirth.

Some childbirth educators have wanted to avoid the word

"pain" so that their students would not be afraid of childbirth. Fear *does* exaggerate the experience of pain. But misrepresentation is not the best way to deal with the problem of fear in childbirth. In the seventies some women used the word "rush" to describe labor pains. The word does approximate the sensation and intensity of a "good" (that is, effective) contraction, but it has not gained general use. Something very dramatic is happening; it may or may not be experienced as painful. Everyone agrees that it is intense and uncomfortable.

A woman's reaction to the discomfort of childbirth will reflect the values of her culture and her feelings about the expectations of others. Some cultures praise a woman for being stoical; others expect her to display terror and anguish. The medical culture of early-twentieth-century America seemed to want to protect women from any sensations or memories of the event. Today, some attendants make a woman feel secure by being responsive to her concerns while giving her the sense that she can do it; others make her feel as though she will not get help unless she is desperate, that she is supposed to "tough it out." If a woman is afraid that the people around her might not respond when she asks for help, she may escalate her reaction to test the caregivers and convince them of her needs.

The modern medical profession was not the first to place its own theories and techniques ahead of the delivering woman's wishes or well-being. In the past, professional midwives often imposed their own myths and practices on the frightened young mother-to-be. Too often, this included strenuous pushing and prodding of the stomach in the belief that the midwife must force the baby's head against the mouth of the uterus in order for the cervix to open. The behavior of midwives was often so strange and occult that, throughout the Middle Ages and into the Renaissance, they were regarded as witches. A midwife wrote a pamphlet that sounded like an early *Thank You, Dr. Lamaze* warning:

Let nature alone to perform her owne worke, and not to disquiet women by the struggling, for such enforcements rather hinder the birthe than any waie promote it.[3]

Fifty years ago, only a little over 50 percent of births in the United States were conducted in a hospital setting. Before that time, midwifery and home delivery by general practitioners were common practice.

In the first half of the twentieth century, the medical profession standardized the procedures the expectant mother must face in the hospital during labor. Some of them, such as the traditional "prep" of the perineal shave and enema conducted in isolation from the husband, are no longer as rigorously enforced as they once were. Others, such as meticulous cleanliness of the staff, intermittent rectal or vaginal examinations of the mother, and the presence of emergency equipment in the room, are still held to be important to the survival of mother and child.

Medical scientists have reason to be proud of the advances they have made in assuring the survival of babies and their mothers. It is no cause for wonder that obstetricians do not hesitate to take the responsibility of childbirth upon themselves and away from the mother and her family. They can provide a sterile environment, anesthetics, and proper instruments to employ in case of complications, all of which are impossible (or at least expensive and difficult) to provide at home.

At the beginning of the fifties, women were almost totally dependent on the new technology of anesthetics and instruments and on the benevolent (male) authorities who wielded them. Most women were unconscious when their babies were delivered. The daughters of these women were left without any tradition of experienced older women who could explain the frightening unknowns of childbirth. With the advent of local anesthetics and movement away from "twilight sleep" and other total anesthetics used in the mid-twentieth century, the childbirth movement became a significant social force. While sometimes referred to as "natural childbirth," it was actually a consumer-based movement that urged obstetrical reform with a preference for "awake and aware" childbirth and family-centered care though it did not insist on nonmedicated births. During the baby boom, so many babies were being born that hospital staffs were stretched to care for them all. Obstetrical care was necessarily impersonal. During the birth dearth of the seventies, hospitals began vying for patients and became more responsive to consumer demands. The childbirth movement, combined with the women's liberation movement of the sixties and seventies, challenged medical authority and helped to humanize birth even in the hospital setting. Partners became an important part of prenatal care. Family-centered childbirth finally caught hold.

By 1990, the issue of childbirth in America seemed to polarize women into those who hoped to bypass all medical interventions and those who wanted the doctor to get the child out as quickly and as painlessly as possible.

The 1980s saw a sharp increase in the rate of cesarean sections. While there is an important consumer movement to try to counter the trend and active associations for VBACs—the catchy phrase that means *vaginal birth after cesarean section*—we must also acknowledge that there is active consumer pressure *for* cesarean sections. Some women would prefer to be delivered surgically rather than face the discomfort of labor. We have returned to a situation reminiscent of the Twilight Sleep Association of the early 1900s through which mothers asked their doctors to put them to sleep. We hear of expectant parents pressuring physicians into providing *more* technological interventions.

Perhaps because they can see it through a sonogram, women may expect the doctor to take care of the fetus and imagine themselves as a passive vessel. Some families seem to believe that the cesarean section is safer for the baby. They hear that babies delivered by c-section are beautiful because they have not been pushed against the birth canal. They hear that cesarean sections are performed because the baby was in distress and the doctors wanted to get it out immediately. It is not surprising that women may believe a cesarean section is the safest route out for the baby and easiest for themselves.

Studies of cesarean section rates show great differences from hospital to hospital and from practice to practice. Private patients in some hospitals are at greater risk for cesarean section than those being cared for in a clinic. It is not clear why. An important factor may very well be that the clinic patients are delivered by house staff, residents who are on duty at the hospital all day and all night and who are salaried, so they do not have the pressure of patients waiting at the office; of additional money to be made from finishing up one case and getting on with another; or the personal pressure of a party to get to on time. We know more operations are performed on Friday afternoon when tired doctors are eager to get home for the weekend.[4]

Obstetricians today expect to be involved in a lawsuit at least once in their career. They know perfectly well that tragedies will occur regardless of technological advances. The best obstetrical care in the world cannot prevent all genetic defects or other flukes of nature. And when there is brain damage or fetal death or extreme maternal distress, in our current culture someone will suggest a lawsuit. Even if the parents are not angry at the doctor and do not blame him, a lawsuit may seem a reasonable recourse to help allay the extreme expense of a damaged child. Other times, of course, the suit is the product of anger. No matter why the suit is filed, the court of law wants to hear that the obstetrician has done everything in his or her power to prevent the tragedy.

A cesarean section is one recourse. Did the doctor perform one? Did he or she perform one in time? Unfortunately, any intelligent doctor following the course of a slow or difficult labor will be influenced by an awareness of the possibility of a lawsuit as he or she follows the progress of a labor and decides how to handle it. We seem to have reached a situation in which considerations that would seem to have very little to do with childbirth are actually controlling obstetrical decisions.

Many doctors try to assure the benefits of family-centered childbirth even with the surgical procedure, allowing husbands to be not only labor support but present in the operating room for a cesarean that may be performed with local anesthesia and the mother awake. They try to minimize separation from the baby; when the mother can't be with the newborn, the father is encouraged to stay with it. Sometimes fathers bond during the early hours that they remain the primary parent or during the weeks when the mother is recuperating from her operation. Both mothers and fathers tend to describe the childbirth experience more negatively if they've had a cesarean section, but there seems to be little negative impact on parental behavior or on self-esteem after the operation. At a 25 percent rate, a cesarean has become a normative experience of childbirth. When handled well, it can be a psychologically positive experience of mastery for a new mother.[5]

The environment and the attitudes of the woman must be appropriate to the kind of labor that is encountered and the kind of care received. A home delivery may be safe and psychologically beneficial to someone frightened of hospitals, but could be disastrous in the case of a cerebro-pelvic disproportion or in the presence of a very anxious father. Any woman who has her heart set on natural childbirth will need emotional support if, for some reason, her condition requires that she have a cesarean. On the other hand, a woman who has counted on having her doctor take care of everything might find herself delivering precipitately at home and be unequipped, emotionally and physically, to handle the situation. Ideally, a woman should be intelligently informed about delivery, be aware of techniques to deal with discomfort, and be in harmony with the people who will be present during her labor. A trusting relationship with the doctor or midwife who will be in attendance goes a long way toward helping a woman feel that the intrusions of birth, like the entire invasion of pregnancy, is a nurturant rather than an assaultive act. She will be able to relax and open herself to the experience.

If a woman feels neglected, persecuted, or ill-used at any time during hard labor or while giving birth, she may be thrown off stride, and her experience of the early hours with the baby may be seriously marred. She may feel too angry, too inadequate, or too frightened to focus on the next stage, that of caring for the infant. But if she feels proud, competent, and trusting through labor and birth, she will be more likely to experience motherhood as a joy. When she is loved and well attended during the birth, a woman starts her maternal experience with a profound model of good mothering. She wasn't protected from all the normal difficulties of life, but she was helped to find her own strength and her own competence.

From the *psychological* point of view, there can never be a "correct" style of coping with labor and birth. The individual life-style of each person and the expectations that one brings to the particular birth environment are the key variables in determining what will be most adaptive. Different labors present different stresses, both physical and psychological, and each woman and couple will respond to these stresses in their own way.

THE EXPERIENCE OF GIVING BIRTH

The physical event of giving birth is tremendous and unforgettable, often much more intense than a first-time mother expects. Childbirth forces a woman to participate in an extraordinary phenomenon which is infrequent in the life of any one woman and much more dangerous than most "normal" life events.[6]

Consider the experience: A mature woman, used to regulating her own life, suddenly finds herself in the grip of an autonomous, uncooperative organ, the uterus, which rises up and performs on its own, almost in spite of anything she may contrive to do for or against it. Her conscious and unconscious wishes hardly matter. It seems out of her control.

This loss of control is the most important psychological aspect of labor for many women. They have to face the reality that they are into something that will simply *happen, with or without their help.* Sometimes labor is fairly easy, sometimes extremely complicated, but universally, the uterus contracts and contracts and contracts, starting slowly and building to a crescendo, following its own rhythms. Doctors can inhibit it temporarily or speed it up considerably. Women can relax and let it flow over them or tense up and fight it. But these factors hardly matter, except as they alter the *experience* of the event. Contractions continue, and the baby exits. If not, the mother's life and that of the baby hang in the balance.

Almost all automatic body functions go on outside of our awareness. Every once in a while they demand our attention, but even then, except for the occasional yogi who devotes his life to learning how consciously to alter a few of them, they are beyond our conscious control and influence.

Most women are sensitive to the functions of the uterus

and the vagina before labor begins. They have probably experienced cramps of one severity or another at some time during menstruation, and certainly have had to be aware of the monthly blood flow. Since the sixth month in pregnancy, they have felt preliminary Braxton Hicks contractions, reminding them once again of the autonomy of the uterus. The vagina, too, has previously gone through its own series of rhythmic contractions in orgasm. The pleasure of these more or less involuntary spasms makes the loss of control insignificant for most women, and may even add to the ecstasy for some. A few women feel something akin to panic at their first orgasm because they may have been unprepared for the brief, intense, and uncontrollable feelings that engulf them. Here, as in labor, there is little possibility of halting the rhythmic contractions once they have begun.

Most women find the comparison between orgasm and labor a dubious one. Even the most devoted followers of "childbirth without pain" movements will not claim that contractions are intensely pleasurable, although there are some women who may draw this analogy with the expulsion of the baby. Nevertheless, the comparison is more easily made by involved observers of the labor experience. A husband who kept a careful notebook while watching his wife in her first labor made this observation: "I keep thinking over and over that there is something positively orgasmic about the contraction—a strange, solitary, almost sexual experience."[7] There are few other physiological events that, once begun, are automatic, involuntary, and take such complete control of all sensations.

The primary biological phenomenon of labor and delivery is determined by the complicated and little-understood physiology of the uterus. The experience of labor and delivery, however, is much more than the simple perception of the strength and duration of each contraction. Whether or not they have read books or taken courses, all primiparas are facing the unknown. Even multiparas cannot predict the course of any particular labor. At a time when so much of her world, even her body image and her life-style, seems out of control, a woman may focus on labor as the central concern in her life. Her body is about to do something on its own, in its own way. What can she do in anticipation of the event? How can she prepare herself to handle it?

The same labor might be experienced as fine by one woman and torturous by another. Some women want very much to have a good birth experience; others don't care at all about how their body performs in labor or expulsion. Personal and cultural values profoundly affect the woman's perception of the event.

Like puberty, marriage, and death, childbirth is one of the great mysteries of the life cycle. The arrival of the newborn may temporarily overshadow the memories and sensations of the birth, but the new mother's perception of her performance and the care she received have great significance for her future female identity and her future relationships, particularly with her husband and children. Birth becomes an opportunity to exercise or learn a coping style that will influence other life situations; that is why it is important for the woman to give birth in a social system that fits her values and expectations and hopes for herself.

Some women spend weeks, even months, learning conditioning techniques for inducing a state that promises to minimize bodily discomfort and to allow maximum active participation in the expulsion of the child. Others react by denying the inevitable experience to the last minute, remaining purposely ignorant of what will happen to their bodies once labor begins. Still others make arrangements ahead of time for a socially convenient day and hour, and rely on the magic of supermedicine through a planned artificial induction or even a cesarean section. Most women avoid these extremes; they have some rudimentary knowledge of what to expect, come to the hospital with labor already in progress, cooperate with the staff in all of their suggestions, and depend on their doctor or midwife to select the most appropriate method of handling the birth.

THE STAGES OF CHILDBIRTH

Labor and birth may sound like simple and predictable events, especially in retrospective accounts. In real life, they are much more confusing. Surprisingly, one of the most anxious times *precedes* the actual labor. Everyone has heard of "false labor," of women who go to the hospital only to be sent home again, but few of us realize how common this experience is. Multiparas go through it more than primiparas. Regular contractions at fairly close intervals may become so much a part of a woman's life in the last few weeks before delivery that she is afraid to believe it is real when labor actually begins. In describing the experience of labor, one woman began with her anxieties during the ten days prior to the birth. In her mind, these days were all part of the labor—and unquestionably the hardest part.

Once labor begins, it follows a predictable sequence from the dilation of the cervix through the expulsion of the new baby.

Medical convention divides labor into four stages. The first stage, dilation of the cervix, begins with the first contractions and lasts until dilation is complete (ten centimeters). This stage is one continuous physical process, but it is divided into three parts that are experienced as very different from each other. The *latent* phase of the first stage extends from the first contractions until the cervix is approximately three centimeters dilated. While there is great variation in the duration of this stage, it averages about eight hours for first-time mothers and about five for experienced mothers. The *active* phase of the first stage is from approximately three centimeters to eight centimeters dilated. *Transition* is the name of the final phase of the first stage, the period when the cervix is dilating the last two centimeters to the beginning of the second stage.

The second stage, expulsion, extends from complete dilation of the cervix until the baby is born. The third stage, placental expulsion, lasts from the birth of the baby until the placenta is expelled. The fourth stage, recovery, lasts from the delivery of the placenta until the mother's physical condition stabilizes.

A perfectly normal labor can last anywhere from two to twenty-four hours. Although the sequence is predictable, the actual nature of the progression through the events is not. Like pregnancy, labor is unique each time. Also like pregnancy, it is possible to sketch a psychological timetable that underlies the labor process. Of course there are exceptions, but we can approximate a description of many women's experience. We must keep in mind that many factors, such as pain-reducing medication, various types of anesthetics, the hospital treatment assumptions, medical interventions (such as fetal monitors or episiotomies), individual psychological differences of the woman and her attendants, and medical complications, may profoundly alter any "general" description.

The first stage, latent phase

The first stage of labor is dilation; the cervix, located at the mouth of the uterus, must be stretched open by the muscular contractions of the rest of the uterus. These are the contractions that take up most of the time of labor for most women. A primipara is likely to be pleased and excited, because she feels that "this is it," and it probably isn't as difficult as she had expected. The light contractions feel substantial, but not overwhelming. Breathing exercises are so effective in dispelling the minimal discomfort that a false sense of optimism may develop. For the more experienced multiparas, these contractions will remind them of what previous labors were like. They may become increasingly anxious as the level of discomfort increases and memories of more difficult stages become distinct. Or they may have heard that second and later deliveries are easier than the first, and feel that this is going to be one of those mythical easy labors in which the cervix opens almost unnoticed and the baby passes through the birth canal before the hospital staff can even whisk the mother into the delivery room.

Some women prefer to be at home as long as possible during the latent aspect of the first stage of labor, especially if the hospital provides nothing but sterile white walls and a narrow bed and expects the patient to remain confined after she is admitted. The time may pass more quickly if the woman is active, perhaps performing light household tasks, reading, or talking with a supportive husband or friends. Rest may be a critical factor, particularly for a primipara who must look forward to hours of labor. Sleep deprivation is a most common complaint in later stages. But a woman must be relaxed and comfortable in order to sleep well without medication. Some women feel most relaxed when they are in the hospital. Others prefer to walk with their partner—stroll in a park adjacent to the hospital, sit in the car watching a sunset. In optimal circumstances, the birth environment will provide a comfortable setting where the mother can feel relaxed and receive intimate comfort from her friends. More comfortable and natural surroundings tend to decrease pain just as much as Demerol at this stage.

Some women are interested in getting to the hospital as soon as possible, so that they can settle in before labor begins in earnest. Watching the nurses bustle about, listening to the sounds of other women, and hearing the occasional wail of a new baby may interest and delight women who can feel themselves part of the dramatic world of a modern hospital. Many women have no strong feelings about where they want to be at the onset of labor. They are simply confused about what is happening and don't know what to do; they tend to want to be in a place where someone will know what to do for them, and so go quickly to the hospital. Much will depend on their feelings about the physical and psychological comfort of the birth environment.

The first stage, active phase

Sooner or later, the more difficult active phase will begin. Contractions will occur more frequently and last longer. Relaxation will become a challenge, even to a trained or experienced woman. Backache, menstrual-like cramps, and fear may become problems, even for a woman who, an hour earlier, had been saying, "Childbirth without pain? Oh, yes, this isn't so hard." This is when the strategies learned in childbirth preparation classes will be put to use and when nursing support and coaching have the most profound effect on a woman's experience. Pain will become an issue. The meaning of the pain for the woman will influence whether or not she will benefit from medication.

If a woman has a high tolerance for pain, she may be thrilled to be able to feel exactly what is happening in her body. For her, it may be intense sensation rather than pain. If she has a low tolerance for pain, she will be happy to accept medication rather than suffer unnecessarily. Hopefully, a woman will react realistically in relation to her own experience and not become trapped by an ideology inappropriate to her.

Some women become extremely bitter about "natural childbirth" indoctrination because it leads them to believe that they are "failures" if they accept medication. This conflict between asking for help versus "toughing it out" may itself add to the discomfort and increase the chances that a woman will need medication. For example, Dahlia suffered intensely through a complicated delivery without drugs. Subsequently, she resented her child and became extremely depressed. Her second delivery was conducted with an epidural anesthetic and left her proud and happy that she had done it the right way—for her.

Medical practitioners continue to debate the advantages and disadvantages of various interventions. In *The World of the Newborn* Daphne and Charles Maurer clearly state that

> if a mother in childbirth receives *any* of the drugs commonly given, then her baby is likely to be born in some kind of drug-induced state and to remain in such a state for days thereafter . . . the baby will not act entirely normal. [8]

Babies, like mothers, are generally resilient and recover from medications appropriately administered during labor or birth. The physical stress of normal contractions actually seems to be good for the fetus. Babies who have experienced some labor breathe more deeply than those who are delivered by cesarean section and go through no labor.

> Apparently, being squeezed toward and through the birth canal squeezes out some fluid that the fetus has in his lungs, enabling the baby to breathe more easily. This is no minor matter, for problems in breathing are a major cause of newborns' sickness and death. [9]

Too much labor, however, can exhaust the baby just as it exhausts the mother.

Sometimes a woman feels that childbirth creates an opposition between her needs and the baby's needs. She may fear that the people taking care of her would save the baby before they would save her. This fear is rooted in a deep, internal struggle. A woman wants to love her baby and do what is best for it, but at the height of a difficult labor, the greater need may be for immediate relief. The baby does not exist for her at that moment. A little reassurance can go a long way, not only to relieve pain but also to relieve the guilt of feeling so selfish just when she is supposed to become a mother, the image of selflessness. Choices around pain medication and other medical interventions have to take both parts of the mother-infant system into account.

Not uncommonly, progress stops, suddenly and mysteriously, somewhere along the way. Contractions may become sporadic after they have been exceedingly regular. When labor slows down or stops, the woman stares at the clock and tries to predict the hour at which she will hold her baby in her arms. She may suddenly experience again the fear that perhaps her body can't do it. Or perhaps she was wrong in estimating her time for delivery. Maybe she'll have to go home and wait some more, when she was so sure that the baby was almost here. If she is weak from hunger and lack of sleep, she will be all the more discouraged and demoralized.

A fresh presence can activate a halted labor. So can a fresh attitude among the people already present. An exhausted woman might use the time to sleep, preparing for the next onslaught. A well-rested woman will benefit from a walk or a shower or a long, luxurious massage. Primitive cultures and modern medicine alike often resort to special potions to stimulate contractions. Enemas, nipple stimulation, rupture of membranes, herbs, and Pitocin are just a few of the stimulants that have been used. A hospital in Scotland has radically reduced cesarean rates by appointing a physician in charge of "active intervention," by which they mean a consultation among the attendants and a discussion of the situation so that the woman in labor is not allowed to lapse into a demoralized state.[10]

A woman's words during labor may give clues about an unconscious process that may be hindering the progress of the birth. For example, a woman might say, "I don't know if I can hold on much longer . . ." She means that she is trying to endure the pain without asking for medication, but the physiological process of "holding on" is antithetical to the process of giving birth. One must "let go," "give in," "enter into the heart of the pain," as a midwife in the Yucatan told her clients.[11] It is not the woman's suffering that helps the baby. On the contrary, the baby benefits from being born into the arms of a secure woman who feels protected, valued, nurtured, and well cared for. All of us flourish in a family that has an emotional economy in which there is enough nurturance to go around.

During the height of labor, the inner world and the outer world seem unusually linked. Looking at flowers opening, thinking of dilation, visualizing orifices of all kinds seem to encourage progress at this stage. Experienced labor nurses tell a woman to stretch her mouth open wide, too. Folk custom in one Indian village recognizes the importance of the symbol of openings. When a baby is being born, the people in the compound loosen their clothing, open doors, and unleash animals to expedite the delivery. As a result, a calf, water buffalo, chicken, or dog may wander into the birthing room and the woman's attendants must chase them out, but this, too, may be seen as a symbolic enactment of the birth process and encourage the baby's exit.[12]

Generally, the rhythm of contractions will continue and accelerate one way or another. A woman may have a desperate realization that now, more than at any other time in her pregnancy, she is trapped in the irrevocable process, that now she is being carried along against her will by a runaway organ. At some point during this long first stage of labor, her membranes will rupture. For many women, this is a particularly regressive phenomenon, for the sudden gush of warm water is reminiscent of wetting the bed during early childhood. The subsequent leaking may continue to be embarrassing.

For the laboring woman, the moments toward the end of the first stage of labor may seem endless. She may find herself wishing fervently for change, wishing for it to get worse so that it will be closer to being over. Even if she has been through it before, she may forget that these feelings are an indication that she is on the brink of change. For this is the phenomenon called "transition" which marks the shift from dilation to expulsion, from stage one to stage two. Contractions may become suddenly different and seem unpredictable, because something new is occurring. The cervix has finished its job. It is open. The baby is starting to move through it, but is not yet fully into position to be pushed out.

The first stage, transition phase

The psychological changes around the time of transition are almost as typical as the physiological ones. Women seem to lose their faith in those helping them. Nothing anybody says or does pleases them. They feel isolated, irrationally angry, and above all, suspicious. "Why am I being examined so frequently?" "What are they all smiling about?" "Why are they all so callous?" "Why don't they listen to me?" At worst, these feelings can be described as paranoid.

These emotional changes during transition are best understood as projections, as casting blame on the outside world for the turmoil and unpatterned feelings that the woman is experiencing inside. The contractions may seem impossible to control. The sensations in the uterus have shifted, so that a woman may fear that something is going wrong, and *nobody seems to understand.*

We once observed an extremely smooth labor of a multipara for whom everything was going well. The staff was fully cooperative and relaxed, warm and encouraging. The woman herself had very good tolerance for pain and was well trained both in breathing and relaxation techniques. Although she reported experiencing discomfort, she gave no outward signs of having any difficulty throughout her first stage. Then suddenly she began to worry. Although she did not seem to be in trouble, she talked about being afraid. The staff knew that she was fully dilated and were enthusiastically preparing for the move to the delivery room, unconcerned by the woman's complaints. When the time came for expulsion, the woman was again optimistic and cooperative. After the birth she said that she had had a burst of irrational anger at her husband, the doctor, and the two nurses. Everybody seemed so excited and happy, so involved in making preparations for the delivery; they seemed to have forgotten about her, to have overlooked the fact that *she* was suffering. In fact, the woman had been attended constantly. She had help through each contraction, both for her breathing and for emotional reassurance. Yet she still felt the overwhelming need to search her environment for the cause of her intense confusion and pain. She did have the realistic fear that if this stage had continued, or had grown worse, she would have been acutely uncomfortable. Physically, she could neither lie still nor get gratification from pushing. She was trapped in the moment, unable to look forward to the immediate future, to some relief. In fact, of course, she was able to push on the next contraction. The baby's head had slipped through the cervix; she had already moved into the second stage.

Happily, the transition phase is relatively brief. It truly is a transition, and the physical demands on the mother change from one kind to another. During the dilation stage, relaxation seems to be the best way to help physiological events proceed as quickly as possible. Suddenly that stage is over and a deeply relaxed woman needs to become alert and energetic to force the movement of the baby down the birth canal. A different order of cooperation is required of her. Everyone in the environment shifts from calm to active as a surge of adrenaline energizes her to the new task at hand.

Even women who have been well prepared for childbirth may be startled by the sensation that occurs as the baby's head turns the corner at the mouth of the uterus and moves toward the opening of the birth canal, for it is not only in the vagina but also in the hip joints. During the pregnancy, ligaments and muscles have loosened to allow greater movement; this process was in preparation for the moment when the baby must slide out. Just as the vagina lubricates during sexual arousal, so, too, it lubricates during childbirth to help the baby slip out more easily. The bones, also, are responding to unusual physiological changes. There is a moment when the woman cannot believe that her body can do it; she has never before felt her bones being pushed apart from within. But if she relaxes and trusts herself, she will discover that her pelvis can yield and spread and make way for the baby to come through. Many women describe the shock of feeling as though they will split open; they don't. They spread and then return to shape.

When transition is over, even the form of the contractions has changed. The baby is no longer restricted to the uterus. It has moved its head through the dilated cervix and entered the birth canal. The crown of its head is visible to anyone who makes an internal examination. The shape of its buttocks are apparent to the mother, who will feel the outline of a different body part each time the uterus clamps down on the baby's body and pushes it farther out. And she will now have the gratifying permission to push, to help with her abdominal muscles and to add a satisfying purposefulness to the automatic contractions of the uterus.

The second stage

The second stage of labor is expulsion. This more than any other time is the work of labor. To a spectator, the grimaces that accompany the necessary pushing may look like pain, although the woman may insist afterward that she did not experience any. Many natural-childbirth advocates remind skeptics that the face of an athlete in competition may also look agonized. Grunts and screams that may accompany the pushing can cause distress among staff and, particularly, among other women in early stages of labor who overhear them. There is no evidence, however, that there is any relationship between the amount of noise and the amount of pain experienced. One patient described her effort to please the staff by remaining calm and quiet; her husband could sense her stoical discomfort and told her to scream if she wanted to. When she finally went ahead and emitted the awful groans that were welling up inside of her, the relief was immediately visible. They seemed to help her push more effectively and gave expression to the ecstasy she was experiencing as she strove to bring forth her new son. As she said afterward, "It wasn't *comfortable*, of course, but the word 'pain' just doesn't seem quite right. It was beyond that. My whole body and mind were into it, and it was intense beyond anything I've ever even imagined."

Anatomical factors seem critical in determining the experience of the expulsion phase. A six-pound baby may slide comfortably through the birth canal of a generously proportioned mother, while a nine-pounder has to be pushed slowly out of a smaller woman. Expulsion of a breech baby may require exquisite cooperation between a woman holding back on her natural impulse to push and the doctor or midwife's delicate maneuvers to control the descent of the baby. The joy experienced in the expression of absorbed work-sounds in a fully alert woman pushing out a well-positioned baby may be very different from the poised control of a delicate delivery, yet both experiences can enhance the self-esteem of the woman who participates actively in the birth of her own child.

Women vary in the degree to which they can tolerate pain and also in their ability to actively push the baby out. Jeanette cooperated effectively during the first stage of labor and was able to relax deeply while listening to her husband's coaching. But when she was fully dilated and it was time to push, she was afraid that the action would make things more painful. She did not want to move into the second stage of labor. She told us afterward that she had the fantasy that if she just continued to be passive, someone else would have to get the baby out. Once she actually got past that resistance and pushed, she found that it was less painful because she could feel that the baby was really on its way.

Some women may want to get through delivery as quickly as possible because they are totally preoccupied with the baby. They describe first *knowing* the new baby in the fullest sense as it moves slowly through the birth canal, the vaginal muscles outlining a large skull, slim shoulders, and brawny torso.

It is hard to evaluate these various feelings. Do they reflect the final fantasies of separation? Are the physical sensations really so acute? One woman described the rhythmic up-and-down, push-and-relax descent of the head as intensely sexual, culminating in the gratifying climax as she finally expelled the baby. Whatever their objective value, these descriptions emphasize the meaning that is intrinsic to the moment of birth.

The third stage

This moment, however, is not the end of the delivery. The afterbirth must be expelled, and if there was an episiotomy (a small cut in the opening of the vagina to eliminate the possibility of tearing as the baby emerges) it must be sewn. Now that the baby is out, a local anesthetic can be used without worrying about it getting into the baby's system. If need be, drugs are given to the mother to decrease any chance of uterine bleeding and promote rapid healing. Mucus is sucked from the baby's mouth to help it breathe. The infant is examined and cleaned by the doctor and nurses. At this stage, the medical people have a lot to do, and the mother, after being the center of attention for so many hours, and after concentrating on her own body and the mysterious movements within it for nine months, may be left alone. Suddenly she has become merely a supporting actress for her squawling hero. This is the moment when a loving friend will be most appreciated, someone who remembers that while newborn infants are terribly important, newborn mothers are important too.

The fourth stage

Fortunately, most births are now arranged so that the mother can make intimate contact with her baby as soon as possible. The philosophy might be articulated as "Take good care of the mother, and she will take better care of the baby." Since the important research findings on maternal infant bonding by Kennell and Klaus in the early seventies,[13] people have been aware that the old-fashioned hospital practice of taking the baby to the nursery as soon as it was born was disruptive, unpleasant, and unnecessary when the mother was awake and alert while her baby was born.

As we are learning so much more about fetal conscious-

ness and newborn competence, we are seeing that a baby
does not simply materialize at birth. It has been with its
mother for months. The relationship has been evolving.
Some women are too concerned about other things to pay
much attention to the baby right away, but most are curious
to see and touch the tiny being with whom they have been
so intimate for so long. And the newborn (if unmedicated)
is alert and awake and curious to smell and nuzzle and
explore.

Healthy humans will learn to love their babies even if
they are separated from them for hours or even days or
weeks (as can happen when a baby is born prematurely).
We can love infants that are not "ours," or infants that
become "ours" even though we did not carry them in our
womb. As psychologist Aidan MacFarlane has said, bonding
is like a courtship. "One can go wrong in different places
and can compensate for it."[14] There is no irreversible magic
in infant-maternal bonding, but the whole point of birth
has been about getting a baby, and once it's there, it's nice
to get a chance to really examine it!

Occasionally a woman will ask to see the placenta. (It is
an extraordinarily beautiful organ; we know one woman
who kept the nurse and baby waiting while the scientific
mysteries of the placenta were explained by the eager obstetrician, delighted at his rapt audience.) But for most
women, the separation from their child, which can last as
long as ten minutes, is a time of anxious expectancy. The
look of joy as a woman is finally allowed to see and touch
her new infant is generally the most emotional moment of
the delivery.

What is she thinking and feeling at this time? Probably
a confused mixture of heightened emotions. She is seeing
a stranger for whom she is supposed to feel all motherly
emotions, a stranger whom, paradoxically, she has known
intimately for nine months. Relief, disappointment, ec-

stasy—it is all here, rolled up in a receiving blanket and placed in her arms. Her body may suddenly shiver in a physiological chill she can't control. Some masked man down between her legs may be stitching her in a most private place. But she is now and forever, indisputably, a mother, the mother of *this* child. No wonder obstetricians say they never get over the thrill of delivering babies. Powerful emotions and mysterious physical events come together in this great crisis, central to our personal experience of life and to the continuance of our species.

The intense ecstasy and vitality frequently experienced in the immediate moments after birth come as a surprise to some women and their partners. Perhaps it is the tradition of hospitalization that leads us to assume that childbirth leaves women wan and exhausted. In fact, even mothers who have gone all night without sleep are apt to have a sudden burst of excited energy. After being tired and enervated through the last few weeks of pregnancy, they seem suddenly transformed, renewed, and radiant.

Twenty years ago, when we wrote the first version of this book, childbirth was just emerging from the closet. There were few descriptions of unmedicated births in American hospitals available for pregnant women to read. The surge of energy that followed the baby's arrival was a great surprise to those who were awake and aware. Now, so many natural and even ecstatic births have been described in popular books that we have heard women express disappointment when they do *not* feel this surge. All we can say is, "Every birth is unique." A woman who does not feel a surge of energy may simply be exhausted from hours of hard labor.

For the medical staff it is all over. The husband may be concentrating on the calls he wants to make to family and friends. An hour after delivery, her baby in the nursery and her husband gone or preoccupied, a woman may be exuberant but empty-handed. She knows that she has entered a new phase in her life, but for the moment nothing has changed except for a strange, empty feeling in her abdomen. It is a difficult moment, and rare for a woman not to experience a slight letdown or even depression as she lies contemplating her future. Whether or not she finds someone to confide in may depend on chance—on whether she is in a single room or has a roommate with values and experiences similar to her own.

Primiparas may be delighted to have nurses handling the baby for them, relieving them of certain feedings, and generally teaching them how to take care of a new infant. Experienced mothers often look forward to their hospital stay with enthusiasm because it is the only time during their childbearing years when they are free from all of their housework and mothering. If they have to resume full responsibilities as soon as they get home, they truly need the days in the hospital. A woman will only look forward to leaving the hospital quickly if she can count on someone—mother, husband, sister, teenage daughter, or professional—to take care of the rest of the family and allow her a few days of bed rest while she gets to know her baby.

Many women leave the hospital within twenty-four hours of the birth. This practice works very well if they will be taken care of at home. The important thing is that they get plenty of rest. Hospitals are not very good places to catch up on sleep!

Labor is a challenging experience even when it progresses smoothly. Women face this challenge in a variety of ways. Some will see it as a peak experience through which they can participate in a major moment of the life cycle and share the bliss and wonder of the newborn baby. Others will see it as a test of personal competence, a challenge of whether or not they can "make it." Some may want to see whether or not their *bodies* can do the job; one woman talked of her "incompetent uterus," which had been unable to perform without the help of inducement through hormones. Still other women may see labor as threatening their identity which may hitherto have been based on the dominance of the will and intellect—faculties that are suddenly forced into a secondary relation to the body and its functions. Almost all women see labor and childbirth as a test of their womanhood. They want to be proud of what has happened.

But different women may be proud of different things; one, of the long name of the fancy anesthetic she was given; another, of the amount of attention from her doctor; a third, of the fact that she did not even once groan or complain; a fourth, that she was able to push out the baby by herself, without anesthetics or instruments.

At the height of labor, a woman must depend on the people surrounding her. Her experience will be radically affected by the amount of security and trust she feels in those elected to help her, by the faith she has in what is happening around her. Unfortunately, a medical ambience imposes definite restrictions on this experience. Most women are more than willing to accept these limitations in return for the safety and the anesthesia that the medical route can offer. But there are women who are willing to do without these advantages in order to achieve their own experiential requirements in childbirth.

BIRTH STORIES

Each birth is unique, and each woman who has given birth finds herself going over the events in her mind for many years afterward. She may discover that the meaning of the experience changes for her over time. It is a major event, one that ushers in a new phase of her life.

The three stories that we have chosen are told by women who had similar expectations. All of them had healthy, easy pregnancies, attended childbirth preparation classes, had an involved partner, established good communication with their obstetrical care providers during the pregnancy, and had a preference for avoiding medications and other interventions during the birth. All three of these women produced healthy girl babies and all enjoyed the early months of mothering.

An easy first birth

Ellen knew something about childbirth because she had visited her older sister in the hospital when she had her babies. Her sister had received an epidural anesthetic for the first birth and had done without for the second. She told Ellen that by the time she had received the epidural the hardest part of labor was over, and she thought "natural childbirth" was much better. Taking her sister's advice, Ellen (and her husband, Ed) interviewed obstetricians to find the one that was best disposed to help Ellen go through labor without medication.

A month before the due date, Ellen and Ed had a serious talk with the obstetrician about medication. Ellen asked Ed and her doctor both to promise that they would not encourage her to "take anything" unless it was medically essential. She wanted very much to try for "natural childbirth." At the obstetrician's recommendation, they called an experienced labor coach and arranged for her to be with them at the birth to help Ellen with pain management and to provide support and explanations whenever they were needed.

When contractions began at eleven in the morning two weeks before the due date, Ed immediately called Cindy, the labor coach. She asked to speak to Ellen and established that the contractions were fifteen minutes apart and not strong enough to cause any change in Ellen's speech or in her breathing. Cindy recommended that both Ed and Ellen rest as much as they could and even sleep if possible. She told them to call back when contractions progressed to five minutes apart.

Ellen and Ed lay down and tried to sleep, but they were much too excited to close their eyes. They had been told that they would probably be up all night and that things could get rough, but as Ellen said, "This is it!" Even though she knew what was sensible, she didn't want to miss a moment of it. She and Ed went out for a long, slow walk.

That evening, Cindy called back. Ed told her that Ellen was still wide awake and that the contractions had picked up and were generally about five minutes apart but sometimes longer. Cindy decided to come over for the night rather than have her sleep disturbed by a call later on. She arrived at about 10 P.M. to find both Ed and Ellen excited at the progress they felt they were making. Ellen wanted to go to the hospital, but Cindy convinced her that there was still plenty of time before the baby would be born. She told them to go to sleep, and she herself lay down on the sofa.

None of them got much sleep. Ellen was too excited to lie down. She paced restlessly. Ed went to bed while Cindy sat up with Ellen. They chatted, took a walk around the block in the moonlight, and practiced breathing exercises. Ellen found that she needed to work with each contraction to relax through it.

At seven the next morning, Cindy called the doctor and told him about Ellen's progress. He told her to take the couple to the hospital and that he would meet them there in about an hour.

By the time she reached the hospital, Ellen was in intense labor. She was glad to lean on Ed to walk from the car to the door and to accept the wheelchair that was provided. Cindy helped with the admittance procedures and knew several of the nurses on duty, which helped keep the atmosphere relaxed and friendly. Ellen was taken to an LDR room, that is, a well-equipped room designed to function for labor, delivery, and recovery. It had all the comforts of home, including a double bed and a rocking chair, but it also contained emergency medical equipment concealed in a cabinet.

When a nurse attached an external fetal monitor, Ellen hardly seemed to notice. She was required to lie down for a half hour while she was on the monitor, but since everything was fine, they removed the monitor and Ellen was again free to move about. She found that she was restless and wanted to pace.

When labor was very heavy and contractions seemed almost continuous, Ellen took a long shower. By ten o'clock in the morning, Ellen felt that she must be fully dilated and was beginning to have some trouble with discomfort, but when the doctor examined her, he found that she was only eight centimeters dilated. This was discouraging news for Ellen.

"I didn't think I could manage it anymore," she told us. "I said I wanted to take something, just to take the edge off so I could get some rest. But they just told me, 'You're doing fine! You don't need anything.' That made me feel horrible. It didn't feel to me like I was doing fine. And then the bag of waters broke. That was the most amazing thing. Labor really changed after that. I had already been tired and having a hard time, but things got more chaotic.

"I became very restless, but the contractions were so hard I could hardly walk. I got out of bed and leaned against the wall. Then I went into the bathroom and I sat on the toilet. At first that seemed to relieve some of the pressure. And all of a sudden I felt like I was going to have a bowel movement. At first I thought that was what it really was, but then I realized that there was nothing in there but the baby! That was what was coming down! I had this terrible fear that the baby would come out into the toilet. I called Ed, who was standing in the doorway. I guess I sounded pretty scared. He and Cindy helped me back to the bed and a nurse checked me. Everybody was amazed and they called for the doctor to come quick! The baby was right there!

"I got scared and again asked for medication. I felt like I was going to split apart. It didn't feel like this could be normal! But Cindy said 'It's too late now. Your baby is right here! Everything is just as it should be. All you have to do is push it out!' I felt disorganized and weird, and scared, too. I didn't know how to get comfortable.

"I'd seen a movie about birthing in a squatting position, and I'd felt better on the toilet than anywhere else, so I asked if I could squat on the bed. The doctor said sure. They had a special pole for me to grab onto. And that is how I delivered my baby: squatting right there on the bed. It was an amazing sensation, and much easier than I expected it to be. It was much easier than the earlier part of labor!"

The baby was healthy and the afterbirth was delivered intact. Ellen was encouraged to breast-feed her daughter almost immediately. Ed went out to phone relatives and friends, but Cindy stayed around for two more hours, until Ellen's mother arrived. Ellen and Ed spent the night in the LDR room, then went home the next day. He stayed home from work for two weeks and Ellen's mother came by every day to help out.

Ellen said that she felt happy about sharing her experience with Ed. She was also glad to have Cindy to talk to. She found herself wanting to tell the story of the birth over and over again in the months afterward. Most people were uncomfortable listening to it, but Cindy always knew exactly what Ellen was talking about and shared enthusiastically in the memories and explained things that Ellen did not understand.

When we asked Ellen how she felt about being turned down in her request for medication, she said, "Oh, they were right! They knew I could do it and they got me through!" She felt her caregivers were following her own instructions to them.

A long, hard labor

Kim assumed she would have an easy birth. She had been very healthy throughout her pregnancy and didn't think she would need any pain relief.

Four days after the due date, Kim woke up at 3 A.M. with mild contractions that were five minutes apart. Nothing seemed to change all day long. She kept in touch with the doctor, who told her to take walks and eat lightly.

At about midnight, the contractions became strong and consistent. Ken called the doctor, who said that if they stayed that way Ken should bring Kim to the hospital in half an hour. But the contractions slowed down until they were fifteen minutes apart again.

Ken was coaching Kim to relax and helped her with the breathing. "He was giving me great moral support. He didn't want me to have any medication. He's against unnecessary medicines and doesn't even use aspirin or cough medicine."

At 4 A.M. the contractions came back up strong and close again, so Kim went to the hospital. She was comfortable with the admission routines of drawing blood and taking vital signs. "But I was put in a tiny little labor room that shared a bathroom with another labor room. Then the nurse came in to examine me and found I wasn't even one centimeter dilated. I felt terrible to hear that, after twenty-four hours of labor!"

The doctor gave her two options: to go home and wait for things to develop, or to stay at the hospital and take morphine to get some sleep. She decided to stay, because she was already exhausted and had hardly begun to dilate.

"Apparently, I slept with the morphine, but it didn't seem like it. I had sort of hallucinations or dreams that I can't remember now, but that were very vivid then." Her husband dozed on a very uncomfortable chair.

At 9:30 A.M. the doctor came, examined Kim, and found she was four centimeters dilated. He broke her bag of waters and found some meconium staining. Because of the meconium, the doctor attached an internal monitor to the baby. Kim was moved to a well-equipped LDR room.

"By noon, I felt really wiped out and was in a lot of pain. I wanted very much to go without medication, but I finally asked for an epidural. The nurse said, 'I know you can do it without it.' Then I asked the doctor and he said, 'Let's try Demerol.' Maybe the Demerol took the edge off slightly but not so that I could notice. I kept waiting for it to kick in, but by three o'clock, nothing. I begged for an epidural. Finally, they called in an anesthesiologist.

"By then I was falling asleep between contractions. I had to sit up for the epidural. For some reason, it took a half hour to administer. My poor husband could hardly stand it. He had to hold me up because I kept nodding off and I was supposed to stay perfectly still for the needle.

"By then I could hardly speak. I had a few words. 'Glasses' meant shove my glasses back up on my nose. 'Drink' meant I was thirsty. My husband was there ready to do what I wanted."

When the epidural started to take effect, Ken went out for a breather, assuming it would be a couple of hours before the final event, but soon after he left, a nurse examined Kim and told her to try to push on the next contraction! Ken came running back in.

The nurse watched the monitor to tell Kim when to push, but she could feel the pressure of the contractions and knew when they were coming. "Then they found that the baby was turned face up. The doctor decided he had to turn her. He tried to do it with his hands, but he couldn't. I heard the clanking of forceps and everybody was rushing all of a sudden and nobody explained anything. They went in with the forceps and turned her. I know I pushed, but I don't remember if they delivered her with the forceps or if they only used them to turn her."

The baby was immediately whisked away to the neonatologist, who sucked out her trachea. "I delivered the placenta and they stitched me up where there had been an episiotomy (which I couldn't feel at all). I was relieved that it was over and I wanted to see the baby. I could hear her but not see her.

"Then they brought her over. It was just overwhelming. Amazing!"

Kim ate a huge meal almost right away and then was moved to the maternity ward. Her baby was born at 6 P.M. on Friday and she stayed in the hospital until 3 P.M. Sunday.

"My husband wanted to get back to his routine to maintain his sanity after all the stress. My mother came on Wednesday and that really helped. I really needed to be in bed and to be waited upon longer than I was. I was exhausted for at least a week."

Kim was left with some difficult feelings about the birth. "I feel guilty about wanting pain relief and the epidural. When I asked for it, I felt they didn't want to hear me. I didn't want to jeopardize the baby with drugs and felt that my husband would think I was 'weak' if I asked. Next time I would go for an epidural right away. If the doctor says to me, 'Let's start with Demerol,' I'll be very clear. 'No. An epidural.'

"I remember how bad it was, but now I have regained my strength and I could go through it again if I had to. It is so rewarding to have the baby. I want another one in two years or so."

Kim's reaction contrasts with Ellen's. Ellen was glad that her caregivers talked her out of medication; Kim wished that hers had provided more, sooner, especially since the baby was in a difficult position. Her suffering did not have any positive meaning for her and contributed to her exhaustion after the baby was born.

A hard labor with problems pushing

Natalie wanted a home birth, but her husband didn't feel secure with that, so the couple elected to go to the hospital and to be attended by a midwife.

Labor started ten days late, a situation that would have been very anxiety-provoking for many women but suited Natalie very well. She and Ned had just moved from another city and were glad to have the chance to settle into their new house before the baby came.

The contractions woke Natalie up in the middle of the night. They were about ten minutes apart. She decided to let Ned sleep until 7 A.M. "I rested between contractions but had to breathe with them. They were manageable because of the time in between."

Natalie called the midwife, who recommended that she stay home as long as possible. Then she called her sister, who had two children of her own and had attended other births. "We hung out at home until three P.M., when my bag of waters broke. Then we went to the hospital. I was five or six centimeters dilated when I got there."

At the hospital, they hooked Natalie up to an external monitor, which she found to be very intrusive. "The monitor had a strap across my stomach and I was used to the freedom of being at home and being able to move around. I said, 'Please remove it.' They said they had to monitor each woman for a half hour when she came in. It seemed like an eternity, it was so cumbersome. I wanted to change positions but couldn't. I don't think it affected the progress of the labor, but it was frustrating and seemed unnecessary."

Natalie's labor progressed smoothly up to pushing. "I never got the desire to push. When the midwife saw that I was fully dilated, she said, 'Okay, why don't you go for it.'

"Maybe it was because I was so in tune with working with the contractions that I didn't seem to want to. There didn't seem to be any reason why I should have pushed so long, for three hours. I could feel when I was being effective and when I wasn't. It was so painful that I would fake it. I couldn't feel where the baby was; by then I was too engrossed in the pain, which was all over, in the back, across the baby, on my belly. Sometimes between contractions it would subside, but it was always lurking.

"At one point when it had been going on a long time, the doctor who is in practice with the midwife was in the room. I was pushing, and he wanted to get on with it. He said, 'Either push this baby out or we'll use some intervention,' meaning forceps or suction. My mild-mannered midwife took him out into the hall. I heard her say, 'Look, she'll push this baby out in her own time . . .'" Hearing him say that made me work harder, because I didn't want an intervention. My husband even said to the doctor, 'Let her do it.' He became my advocate in the truest sense, helping me to do things the way I said I wanted.

"I tried to push, but just wasn't very good at it. I didn't seem in tune with that part. Finally they said, 'Hold back, slow down,' but on the next contraction I pushed anyway— I wanted to go for it. I'd been having such a hard time with the pushing that I just didn't want to hold back anymore. There was a warm sensation, a gush, something warm just sliding out.

"I was too inside the pain to look in the mirrors. Ned was up with me rather than where the action was. They let us do what we wanted to do.

"When she finally came out, I experienced relief instead

of joy. We were both so dazed and stunned. They put her across my chest and finally the midwife asked, 'Would you like to know if it's a boy or a girl?' That snapped me back into reality.

"The baby was lying across my stomach and the cord was still intact, the placenta not delivered. I could tell she was fine because my sister had a glowing look on her face. I was still feeling a little removed from her, didn't sweep her up. But after I really held her, that distance went by the wayside. She wasn't just this being draped across my belly but was Millie, my baby."

Natalie and Ned stayed in the hospital that night and the next. Natalie enjoyed the chance to rest and have three meals a day prepared for her. She found all the information from the nurses very helpful. "Then we spent three days at home, just the three of us. That was a very special time. Then Ned had to go back to work and my mother came to stay with me for ten days.

"I want to have another child. I'd love a written guarantee that it'd be easier. It's scary to me; I've never experienced anything like it, ever, but I'll do it again. I feel badly that I wasn't in tune with the whole part of her arriving and didn't feel the head, the shoulders, and the body delivered. But I did it, and the midwife and my husband and my sister were all wonderful. They all helped me through it, even when I had given up hope. They believed in me. My sister was especially attuned to me. At one point, when the midwife was telling me some story, Jan just said, 'I don't think Natalie is interested in listening to that just now.' And she was absolutely right. I am much too polite a person ever to tell someone I'm not interested in their story, but Jan was able to do it for me. I felt she was right there with me, knowing what was going on inside my body."

In childbirth, the word "easy" is a relative thing. We call Ellen's experience easy, yet her description indicates how

very straining and challenging it was. But she coped well
with the stress. The medical routines did not bother her
and she felt free to experiment with positions that helped
her. She was lucky to have her baby in a good position and
to be able to push effectively.

Fatigue and pain became significant factors for both Kim
and Natalie. Both of them had entered labor hoping not to
use medications or medical interventions. Both had their
caregivers suggest that they change this plan. Because of the
meconium staining, speed became an important issue for
Kim's labor. The doctor could not risk three hours of in-
effectual pushing and used forceps. Natalie had no indication of any problem with the baby, so she was allowed
to continue to try to push the baby out, even when one
caregiver wanted to intervene.

Both Kim and Natalie were left with unresolved feelings
about their experiences. They had had a hard time and
wondered how things might have gone differently. Kim felt
guilty asking for medication. Natalie felt guilty for not pushing more effectively. Months after their babies were born,
they were still attempting to evaluate what had happened
and make good choices about care for their next labor. It
is especially interesting to see that each one felt that the
final choice about intervention was best for her. Kim wants
an epidural sooner next time. Natalie wants to go without
drugs again. Most important, both women have healthy
babies and have become devoted mothers. While the experience of childbirth was important to them, they did not
use it to define themselves as mothers. It was not the keynote
of their relationship to their babies.

Toward the end of their first pregnancies, most women
wonder about pain management during labor and want
reassurance that the people who are with them will be responsive to their needs. Some women are afraid that their
doctors will impose too many drugs or other intervention

on them; others are just as afraid that the doctor will refuse to help them when they ask for assistance. As we can see from the experiences of Kim and Natalie, the concerns are real. It is hard for caregivers to evaluate when to administer pain relief and when to rely on emotional support and encouragement.

The most important tool for pain relief is the trust between the laboring woman and her caregivers. The labor coach, whether it is the woman's partner, her sister, or a professional coach, becomes her advocate when she is in distress. We believe that the greater the understanding and the greater the ability to truly evaluate the laboring woman's needs and desires, even without verbal communication from her, the better the woman will feel about her experience after the event.

5

The Expectant Father's Experience

THIS CHAPTER will attempt to outline the *experiential world* of expectant fathers, much as the earlier ones focused on pregnant women. Our society still does not validate the experiences of fathers-to-be as important or even acceptable. The father's role is often defined as that of support for the mother, an exceedingly important function, but not the whole story. Men experience pregnancy in their own right. Every study of expectant fathers has demonstrated that men go through pervasive psychological changes in the transition to fatherhood.[1]

A man's experience of pregnancy is not triggered by hormonal or bodily changes, but his personal and social transformation may be as great as his partner's. To become a father for the first, second, or fifth time requires a total reorientation of the meaning of his life. Men need the nine months of gestation to help forge their new identity. Too often, they feel left out, as though their needs and changes are irrelevant. The cultural image of the heroic male is still epitomized by the rule of the sea, women and children first. In his role as "captain" of his family, a father may feel that he should stay behind and sacrifice himself for the sake of others. A man may feel guilty and inappropriate for wanting to be saved himself when obviously his wife is the one who is "really" needy. No matter how significant a man's reactions to pregnancy may be, he may feel that his wife is in the throes of such extensive physical and psychological change that he must repress and contain his own experience for her benefit. We believe that his experience of expectant parenthood must be acknowledged and lived out as fully as possible for his own and his family's benefit.

The father as provider

Thirty years ago, when we began studying pregnancy, the popular culture assumed that the father-to-be played a strained and peripheral role during pregnancy and childbirth. One current cartoon showed a middle-class father sitting with his small son, saying, "Mommy's gone to the hospital to bring home another mouth to feed." The basic stereotype was of the husband drinking at a corner bar and handing out cigars while his wife labored alone. The ideal father was a provider, not a nurturer. He went off early in the morning and returned late in the day while the mother stayed home with the children. "Masculine" was conceptualized as distinct from "feminine." There was little men could do to directly involve themselves in pregnancy or childbirth.

When gender roles are rigorously separated, as in the Victorian era and again in the 1950s, men have little involvement with domestic matters. Since the 1960s, traditional gender differences have been challenged. Women still tend to do more housework than men and obviously are still the ones who get pregnant and give birth to babies, but more of the total experience of parenthood is shared.

The involved father

Over the past three decades of increased male involvement in childbirth and in parenting, men are becoming more aware of their own major life transition and seek to have their own personal experience. Now most middle-class fathers-to-be go to at least one meeting with the obstetrician during the pregnancy, attend childbirth preparation classes, learn about labor and birth, and form a relationship with their infants. The change is consistent with our culture's movement toward greater parity between the genders, women's increasing role in the work force, the loosening of rigid concepts of "masculine" and "feminine," and the growing assumption, supported by law in many states, that men can be as well qualified as women to be the custodial parent in case of divorce.

The movement to include fathers in childbirth started when men were the only reliable support for women in our mobile society. In the era after World War II, the extended family was often far away, leaving a young woman without her mother or another close female companion during the childbearing years. During that period, couples married young and had children early. The husband became the prime "mothering" figure for his dependent wife, although he had little preparation for this role.

In most families today, the father is trained to be the mother's coach during labor, helping her learn relaxation methods and special breathing techniques for labor and birth. In this role, he is supposed to take care of everything in the outside world, which gives little validity to any internal experience he might have. Both father and mother may feel that they are uninitiated in the "women's mysteries" of babies or the "medical mysteries" of obstetrics. The typical man has been raised to feel he is not allowed authority in either, even when he is becoming a parent.

Before the pregnancy, particularly the first, he has learned to rely on his wife for support at times of stress. Just when he must cope with her apparently unmotivated emotionality, her physical complaints, her shifting sexuality, and her ever-changing body, she requires extra support, understanding, and consolation. While he is wrestling with feelings about the added responsibilities of fathering, he must learn to "mother" his wife, so that she can feel more comfortable about accepting the changes in her life. All through the pregnancy, his needs are secondary. He may be asked to give up sexual intercourse, to take on extra domestic tasks, even to take on an additional job. If, prior to pregnancy, a large part of the marriage relationship has been based on a maternal wife, he may be faced with a difficult adjustment to her increased inwardness, passivity, and dependence on him.

Running away

Faced with the anxiety of unpredictable change and no direct way to master the experience, some expectant fathers find that they cannot tolerate being in the family. There are many forms of "running away." Often there seems to be an explanation: business trips, new casual acquaintances, ball games. The pattern develops gradually and extends itself into long absences from home or sexual affairs with other women.

A man can choose to disengage himself from the pregnancy process; he can leave his partner entirely, or he can deny that the event has any effect on his psyche or on his responsibilities. But if he does disengage, he may work against the best interests of his family and deprive himself of an opportunity to widen and enrich his own experiential world and begin the psychological preparation critical to becoming a father.

The "running away" reaction interacts with his partner's increased neediness during pregnancy. At first she is likely to feel extremely threatened by her husband's absence; her dependence will increase, and she will be aggravated by his not being there when he is most needed. She may then make the kind of psychological demands that threaten his autonomy and drive him even farther from home. This vicious cycle may eventually cause irreparable damage. Marriages sometimes end under the stress of pregnancy.

One woman told us that she understood what her partner was doing when he took off on a cross-country motorcycle ride. She said, "I'd run away if I could. The problem is, if I ran away, the kid would come with me, right here in my belly." Her partner acted out the fear and ambivalence they both experienced.

Couvade syndrome

It is still rare for a man to admit openly that he is in the midst of a profound emotional experience during his wife's pregnancy. Yet a man's response to becoming a father cannot be neutral. The issues are too large, too meaningful, to be ignored. In fact, whenever men have been the subject of systematic study during their wives' pregnancies, the findings have suggested that major changes are taking place. Several medical researchers have found a statistically higher incidence of physical symptoms among men with pregnant wives than among a matched sample of other men. Men may develop mild physical complaints, bouts of anxiety, or unexplained fears and compulsions during pregnancy. Weight gain, nausea, stomach distress, loss of appetite, toothache, and even abdominal bloating are the most common physical changes. These problems, like the milder symptoms women experience, often alternate with periods of emotional stability and feelings of well-being, and they disappear after the child is born.[2]

These psychosomatic symptoms are called a *couvade syndrome*. Unlike "ritual couvade," an anthropological term for cultural patterns that regulate the various dietary, confinement, or pseudo-labor behaviors for expectant fathers, the changes of the couvade syndrome are psychological, generated from within the man himself, and not social, dictated by the culture. Often they are not consciously perceived by the man and are not recognized as related to pregnancy by the people around him. The physical symptoms themselves *express* the conflicts that are triggered by the pregnancy. Sometimes a symptom may be a simple manifestation of anxiety, as with a husband who always tends to react to tension by overeating and who gains twenty-five pounds during his wife's pregnancy. At other times, however, the meaning of a particular symptom can become much more symbolic, as when a stomach is distended but there is no weight gain. Then the emotional roots are related more directly to deep feelings about the pregnancy, including envy or hostility. Weight gain may express a man's intimate and positive identification with his partner. Similarly, men often dream they are pregnant or have given birth, which may be interpreted as anxiety or envy or may be seen as an attempt to share deeply in the woman's experience.

From anecdotal accounts, it is our impression that troublesome physical symptoms are rarely present in both partners, almost as though a man who is experiencing morning sickness is doing it for his wife. She may be relieved and grateful for his demonstration of involvement, or she may think he is "weird" or, occasionally, may resent his acting as though the pregnancy were *his* when she had been expecting it to be her private experience. Something is growing and changing, but how are men to experience it?

The impulse to find a new and important role in life just when a wife becomes pregnant seems a fairly typical male response to pregnancy, a man's attempt to deal with pressures he cannot quite bring into focus, pressures to experience something like that which his wife is more obviously encountering through her changing body. A new hobby may be an indication that a man is feeling the need to develop a new way of life but has no way to satisfy this urge through direct involvement in his identity as father-to-be.

Margaret Mead emphasized human fatherhood as a social invention. She is obviously correct, since except for the moment of conception, the biology of human pregnancy makes the man superfluous. However much difficulty fatherless children have in psychological and social adjustment (and they do[3]), they develop and emerge from the uterus in much the same way as those children who have the concerned attention of their fathers. Fathers do have a role in child development, but it does not have a biological base as intense as gestation and lactation. It is hard for a human male to know quite what to do to express his transformation into a father. Perhaps the couvade symptoms are an unconscious attempt to deal with that question.

We cannot draw any conclusions about what is natural for humans, for our species always shapes behavior in relation to culture. We do not respond exclusively to hormonal or instinctual patterns. Our temperaments impel us toward parenting, and a man may be as invested in the fantasy of giving birth as a woman. One of the tabloid newspapers recently implied that this had already happened, as its headline screamed that the man in the cover photo had given birth to a daughter. The article was not quite as dramatic as the headline. The story was about a mother who subsequently had a sex-change operation, not about a man who gave birth to a child, but the headline spoke to our fascination with the possibility that a man just might be able to do it.

Ritual couvade

Studies of the expectant father in other societies provide a glimpse into some of the ways fathers *do* experience pregnancy and childbirth.[4] Many customs fall under the general heading of ritual couvade phenomena. *Couvade* is derived from the French verb *couver*, which means to brood or hatch. The term was first used by anthropologists to designate a series of related behaviors involving regulations for the father during the period around childbirth. Frequently, the father is required to observe certain rest patterns, dietary restrictions, and work prohibitions.

In some tribes, the man and woman must both avoid eating the flesh of particular animals whose young are born blind, for fear that the unborn child will also be born blind. A husband in the Ifage, a tribe in the Philippines, is not allowed to cut or kill anything during his wife's pregnancy. This restriction extends to such essentials as cutting wood, forcing his relatives to help him and thus acknowledge his special status. Among the Chaorati, a tribe in South America, the husband must keep to his hammock during and for several days after the delivery. At the time of birth, he mimics the labor and goes through the motions of delivery. The Kurtatchi fathers in the Pacific Islands must stop work and go into seclusion at the time of delivery. They are not permitted to eat certain foods, such as pig, fish, or opossum, and are forbidden to lift anything heavy or touch a sharp object. After the fourth day, they are allowed to meet the new infant and must give him a medicine that is supposed to make him strong. But among the Siriona in Bolivia, the father must go off to hunt as soon as labor begins, and must name the child after the first animal he kills. The mother hopes for the hunter's speedy success, since the cutting of the cord must wait until the husband returns, when he will perform the operation.

Students of these customs, which stress imitation of the

female, feel that they represent a form of the sympathetic magic that is common in many nonliterate cultures. The husband simulates his wife's childbirth or acts like her in the postpartum period in the belief that evil spirits may be fooled into pursuing him, letting the mother and baby live unharmed. More sophisticated cultures may discount this idea as fantastic, and its attendant behavior as unnecessary, but the couvade phenomena have the important side effect of helping a husband play an important part in pregnancy and childbirth and dramatically evolve into a father in the eyes of his wife and society. In addition, they help a man cope with the envy and competitiveness that he may feel at a woman's ability to perform such a fundamental creative act. Lastly, in his activities to deceive the evil spirits, a man may also find a reasonable outlet for his own desire to take on something of the female role in life.

The practices of other cultures do not provide reasonable alternatives for us. Customs function most effectively when they are appropriately adapted to the society in which they are practiced. If in a certain culture the biological father is to have no role in raising his child, there may be no need for him to have any role in its nurture or at its birth. There are cultures that give the husband even *less* of a role than our own. For example, in Japan, where the worlds of men and women have traditionally been kept separate, women often go to live with their own mother near the end of the pregnancy and recuperate there after the birth. Not only is the father not present at the birth, but he

> may or may not visit on Sundays after the baby is born. It is not unusual for the father's first contact to be the day he brings his wife and baby home.[5]

A society may give interesting reasons for encouraging a father to be present at the birth of his children. Anthropologist Brigitte Jordan notes that in the Yucatan, they say he should see "how a woman suffers." This rule is quite strong and explicit and we heard of cases where the husband's absence was blamed for the stillbirth of the child.[6]

Jordan also reports that the husband's witnessing of his wife's pain is used to remind him of the importance of abstaining from intercourse postpartum.[7]

There is no reason why a husband should not cut the umbilical cord of his own child and thereby *actually* participate in the physical separation of the infant from its mother. Similarly, why should the husband not be the central figure for his wife during labor, rather than let a stranger in a green gown take over? Couvade customs serve an important psychological function for the husband and wife. Perhaps our own rituals (or lack of rituals) for the pregnant husband are limiting a potentially rich experiential event or causing harm to the individual and his family. We may be failing to satisfy a man's psychological requirements at this turning point in his life. He is establishing a new relationship with his wife, his child, and within himself.

The little boy's relationship to pregnancy

As has been emphasized throughout this book, pregnancy is more than simply a biological event; it is a time when identities are changing and new roles are being explored; it is a time when childhood fantasies and universal myths are painfully and joyfully close to everyday awareness. The father is not immune to these changes even if he does not have a moment-to-moment physical reminder of them within his body. Unfortunately, in our culture a little boy is rarely as consciously prepared for his future role as father as his sisters are for theirs as mother. No one takes him aside to tell him what to expect at childbirth or during pregnancy. And yet the little boy who still feels intimately, almost symbiotically, attached to his mother cannot escape being influenced by the experience of watching her become increasingly pregnant and of seeing her come home with a new infant. Since he is neither blind to her physical changes nor deaf to her emotional fluctuations, he becomes laden with personal myths that he will carry in his unconscious all his life.

Many little boys believe that they are pregnant at one time or another in their childhood. If their mother's belly can swell and grow a baby inside, why can't theirs? They too have stomachs that change shape as they eat and drink. They too produce feces. Why not something else? By going through the fantasy of being pregnant, they may try to master the mysterious and frightening event they observe in child-bearing women, above all their own mothers.

Psychoanalysts have suggested that the fantasy of pregnancy by oral conception is a normal developmental stage, as true for boys as it is for girls. What differs is the way parents deal with the ideas. When a little girl proudly proclaims that she is pregnant, she is rarely ignored. The tense may be changed; she may be told that she cannot be pregnant *now*, but that she will be some day. Her ability to identify with her mother and with other women will help her gradually to give up the fantasy and be satisfied with the promise for the future. It is not so simple for a little boy.

We knew a two-year-old boy who informed his pregnant mother that he, too, had a baby in his belly. Each day he listened to the explanations that his family offered him about boys and men not getting pregnant, but each day he reaffirmed with great solemnity that he, too, was pregnant. He accepted the fact that he had a penis like Daddy's, and he acknowledged that he would grow up to be a father, not a mother. But he still carried the idea of the baby growing inside of him. Apparently his penis could not compare with the remarkable living protuberance that he saw on his mother, and the role of father did not for him preclude the function of childbearing. The idea went away after the baby was born, but the little boy then desperately wished to be able to nurse the baby, and even offered his own tiny nipples to his little sibling. He tried sleeping in a crib like the baby and sleeping in a big bed like Daddy; but what he most wanted was to be able to be like Mommy. We cannot visualize this little boy twenty years later going through his wife's first pregnancy without experiencing powerful feelings of identification and envy toward his wife. He may deny them and be aware only of a vague uneasiness, a disquiet about his own masculinity and identity. Or he may try to understand them, amplify them, and even revel in them. But he will not be unaffected. On some more or less primitive level, he will reexperience them.

In *Childhood and Society*, Erik Erikson describes a four-year-old boy named Peter who retained his bowel movements for up to a week. He was even able to withstand a large enema meant to relieve his bloated abdomen. Erikson describes his encounter with the boy in his room:

> I admired his books and said, "Show me the picture you like best in the book you like best." Without hesitation he produced an illustration showing a gingerbread man floating in water towards the open mouth of a swimming wolf.
>
> The boy excitedly commented that it wouldn't hurt the gingerbread man to be eaten because he wasn't alive. The next picture he showed was from *The Little Engine That Could*, which showed a smoke-puffing train going into a tunnel and then on the next page emerging not smoking. Then the boy said, "The train went into the tunnel and in the dark tunnel it went dead."[8]

Erikson comments: "Something alive went into a dark passage and came out dead. I no longer doubted that this little boy had a fantasy that he was filled with something precious and alive; that if he kept it, it would burst him and that if he released it, it might come out hurt or dead. In other words, he was pregnant."[9] This boy had been told that he had been too big to come out when his mother sat on the toilet, which was this family's euphemism for childbirth. He had been delivered by cesarean section. A brief description of the anatomy of pregnancy and birth had dramatic results. He soon produced a huge bowel movement.

In cultures where birth takes place at home, children and adolescents observe the activities surrounding birth and grow up with a sense of its difficulty. In such cultures, "children . . . play at having a baby" and "the 'father' takes an active part."[10] Men as well as women carry with them their childhood fantasies about pregnancy. It is difficult to generalize about what specific effects boyhood ideas and experiences will have on the effect of pregnancy on a mature man. One may feel excluded, put down, and unimportant, symbolically castrated at a time in his life when he is expected to assume more masculine roles. Another may feel that he, like his wife, is growing both psychologically, as he becomes aware of the feminine, nurturant aspects of himself, and socially, as he prepares to take on new duties in his life.

Identification with the feminine

Psychologically and embryologically, every man is part woman and every woman part man. Lying next to an ever-changing pregnant woman in bed may be a reminder to a man of his potential to be something new, to grow from inside, to experience rebirth. It may stimulate a reevaluation of the too familiar and fixed image of his own self. One father described listening to a talented musician when his wife was six months pregnant and suddenly being overwhelmingly jealous and feeling a deep and frightening emptiness. He was depressed in the face of the musician's and his wife's creativity. He felt the need to build something, to have something grow under his hands. Dostoevsky's involvement in his wife's first pregnancy was so intense that it pervaded his language as well as his ability to create:

> The idea I have is so good and so pregnant with meaning that I worship it. And yet what will come of it? I know beforehand. I'll work on it for eight or nine months, and I'll make a mess of it.[11]

He had found himself unable to write at all during the first six months of the pregnancy, although his idea eventually produced one of his greatest novels, *The Idiot*.

Pregnancy evokes an identification with feminine aspects in a man's history and makeup which is sometimes awesome and even unacceptable. Some men become impotent at this time, despite the heightened sexuality of their wives and before any major physical changes of pregnancy have occurred. Others may escape into visibly masculine endeavors like fixing cars or playing football. One man became an avid mountain climber during his wife's pregnancy, only to give up the hobby once his baby was born. On the other hand, certain husbands are most secure and sexually active during their wives' pregnancies. A man's reaction is overdetermined by the myriad of factors that have contributed to his personal sexual identity. Pregnancy acts as a stimulant, a reminder of what lies below the tip of the iceberg, that part of the psyche that one hardly knows and rarely needs to face so directly.

Identification with the father

A crucial part of the experience of pregnancy for the man will be his feelings about fatherhood. As we have noted, cultural guidelines for his attitudes and expectations are much more blurred than for the expectant mother. The mother-child relationship has been closely examined by literally thousands of studies, while the father-child relationship has, until the 1970s, been all but ignored, as if the father, either by his presence or absence, did not contribute to a child's development. We have begun to learn how interdependent we are and how "codependencies" can be harmful as well as supportive. We now look at the entire family's contributions to the problems of each of its members. Fathers' contributions to child development and to family dynamics are being studied, particularly in the critical dimension of their absence or their presence.

There are stresses to becoming a father that go beyond present-day role uncertainties or even the economic demands that a new child creates. Impending paternity uncovers all the memories and emotions of what it was like to be fathered as a child. An expectant father named Roger shared his thoughts with us:

> I rethink past experiences with my father and my family and am aware of how I was raised. I just think I don't want to do that again, I want to change that; I don't want to be like my father in that way. I wish there had been more connection and closeness and a lot more respect for who I was. For me, my father-in-law combines spontaneity, sincerity, and warmth. He is a model of that mix of empathy and warmth plus stepping back and being objective that I want as a father.

The primary experience for learning about fathering is the son's relationship with his own father or other fathering figures. The father-to-be may be flooded with forgotten images—playing ball, being tossed into the air, learning how to do household repairs with his father at his side, seeing his father hold him in the mirror and wondering who was who, feeling the living line between grandfather, father, and son, and discovering immortality in a family name or a family nose. Then there are the disturbing residues: loneliness at being ignored by the provider, longing for male contact in a woman-dominated home and school, fear of being hit by a raging giant, or watching, helpless to intervene, as an argument between parents threatens to tear apart the foundations of his universe. To become a father in one's own right, to have a son or daughter oneself, means to take on the role that he had always been free to criticize in his "old man."

Many of these emotions are experienced at a more intense level during pregnancy than in the months and years after the child is born. The impending unknown triggers the dreams and anxieties that are a part of imminent fatherhood. This is especially true for first-time fathers, who may never have thought of themselves as a parent. Once the baby arrives and becomes part of the household, the magic feelings of paternal creation may slip away in routine existence, only to be felt again at such vivid landmarks in a growing father-child relationship as the first time they go to a ball game together or share something special and masculine. The bar mitzvah, high school graduation, wedding, or any other ceremony marking a boy's growth into manhood may also make father and son briefly conscious of themselves as two men at separate stages of the same cycle, one learning to be a man from the other, who may not feel fully competent in manhood himself.

During pregnancy, there is no reality, no child to feed and to help, no really helpless creature to provide for, no one to discipline, to take places, to show off for. There may be little to do but plenty to be anxious about. A man may wonder what kind of father he will become, how he will be accepted, what sort of a model he will provide for a child who may ultimately see through him to the pettiness, the

immorality, and the ego trips. But action is for the moment
suspended in the uncertainty of who the new baby and new
father will be.

Sometimes the question of the gender of the child is a
focus for the prospective father. He may know what a boy's
relationship to a father is like from his own childhood experiences, but he may not be able to anticipate the feelings
of a father toward a daughter. There is a soliloquy from the
musical comedy *Carousel* that describes the reaction of a
pregnant father who feels he must transform his life because
of the possibility of having a daughter. The hero, a carousel
pitchman, has been singing with joy at the discovery of his
wife's pregnancy. He is thrilled about the prospect of having
a boy who *"can call me the old man,"* and of whom he can
be proud, *"the spittin' image of his Dad."* Suddenly he
realizes that he could have a girl, and the tone changes:

> *What if he is a girl?*
> *What would I do with her?*
> *What could I do for her?*
> *A bum with no money.*
> *You can have fun with a son,*
> *But you've got to be a father to a girl.*

Then this expectant father, frightened by the thought of
having a daughter, makes a decision that will eventually
cost him his marriage and his life:

> *I gotta get ready*
> *Before she comes,*
> *And make certain that she*
> *Won't be dragged up in slums*
> *With a lot of bums like me.*
> *She's gotta be sheltered*
> *And fed and dressed*
> *In the best that money can buy.*

I've never known how to get money before,
But I'll try, by God, I'll try!
I'll go out
And make it,
Or steal it,
Or take it,
Or die![12]

Some men want a little girl rather than a boy because of the fear of reexperiencing their own childhood nightmares. This is particularly true of men who grew up without a father or an important male figure in their lives. How can one become a father without knowing what it feels like to be fathered? Some men who never knew their own fathers do not wait to test this challenge, and leave the woman once she is pregnant. The fear of remaining is often expressed as a fear of taking care of the mother and child. It may be initially expressed in terms of financial responsibility—which may be real or a screen for a deeper sense of emotional inadequacy. Underneath the economic fear looms the specter of failure, of being hated by a child the way they themselves hated the man who abandoned their own mother. These men know firsthand the tremendous demands of a little boy on a father who cannot or who is afraid to fill the need. So they, too, leave, perhaps returning home as occasionally as their fathers had before them. And yet the little boy may always be on their minds. Their successes and failures may be viewed in relation to their sons. They fear the boy because they know what he may be thinking.

Ambivalence

Pregnancy can elicit ambivalent feelings even in an experienced family man. It provides a pause in an enforced routine, months to reevaluate what it will be like to be a father of another child, and by implication, what kind of father he has already been to his other children. The weight of responsibility may become increasingly heavy with each pregnancy. Only the man who has a son or daughter can know how deeply a child will affect his inner and outer world. While the fantasies of the new prospective father may rest on unknown and untested aspects of himself, the more experienced father already knows his potential. If he is proud of his prior fathering, and if the new child is wanted, he may experience the most profound ecstasy and fullness during the pregnancy and birth, feeling the joy of being able to create new life, unmodified by the fear of being a failure in the role of parent. One experienced father described feeling pleasure at his own "heaviness." The impending birth of another child made him acutely aware of his bonds to his family. He described the feeling as an "oceanic" one like falling in love, losing himself in the feeling of connectedness and closeness with others. He became obsessed with a Bob Dylan song, "Father of Night," and experienced himself as an all-powerful creator:

> Father of night, Father of day,
> Father who taketh the darkness away,
> Father who teacheth the birds to fly,
> Builder of Rainbows up in the sky,
> Father of loneliness and pain,
> Father of love and father of rain . . .[13]

After the crisis of delivery and the reintegration of the family with its new member, the song passed from his mind. His fathering became again more routine and less miraculous.

Let us look in more detail at a man's interaction with his partner during the nine months of pregnancy. Strictly speaking, he is not on the fixed biological timetable of his wife and does not undergo distinct hormonal changes. Nevertheless, his reactions will be closely linked to her changing form and emotions, and to the approaching day when his child will appear.

As we become more familiar with the ways that men experience pregnancy and paternity, we will be able to help more men participate openly in the unique aspects of these demanding and potentially fulfilling nine months.

THE FIRST TRIMESTER

Readiness for parenthood

Men talk about their readiness for parenthood in terms of personal freedom. They are aware of the financial burdens and social restrictions that come with the role of father, as described by Larry, a commercial artist, who told us, "I knew Monica wanted to have kids and she said it had to be fairly soon. Having kids was fine with me but I had a lot of anxiety about the money. Finally I just thought, 'I'm never going to have enough nuts stored up in the tree. If you're going to have a family, just do it. It will work out.' "

Men wonder if they are "ready to give up childhood" or if they want to "really become a grownup." They fear loss of freedom, loss of independence, and loss of romance with their partner. They may think of the five- or six-year-old child they will gain eventually, but they often have little sense of pregnancy, childbirth, or an infant as positive benefits in their personal lives, even when they are actively involved in the decision to have a baby.

Many men feel pressured to have a baby because the woman wants one. Couples frequently seek counseling around this issue. If the man truly does not want a baby (or another baby, as is often the case when the man has children from a previous marriage), and the woman feels that she must have one to feel she has lived her life fully, even couples who are very much in love sometimes break up.

Sometimes the man is the one more eager to have a child. In Japan the saying that "a woman is a borrowed womb"[14] implies that the father is the important parent; the child is his, even though he does not participate after conception and does little or no child care. Another unusually clear case of the father as the dominant parent occurs when a homosexual man hires a surrogate mother to be impregnated by his sperm with artificial insemination, a true "hired womb," so that he can have "his" child.

Conception

Even when both partners agree to have a baby, a man may feel that he is being used by a woman for impregnation, so that she can have "her" baby. If conception doesn't occur right away, he has to be at the beck and call of his partner and her temperature chart. The situation becomes most obvious in cases of artificial insemination, when pregnancy cannot arise easily out of sexual intercourse and the woman just wants a man's sperm.

Even before pregnancy, a strong marital alliance is a profound asset for the strains of parenthood. As one man told us, "I worry about all the time demands that come with a baby. Even with all the good things we have in the relationship, it is already difficult."

If a man's identity is profoundly linked to the idea of being his father's son and oedipal feelings about competition for the mother have never been comfortably resolved, the idea of impregnating a woman may activate unconscious fears of retribution by the "real" father. For other men, the idea of impregnation adds intensity to sexuality. Many men find even their dreams filled with more sexual activity than usual.[15] The tone of this eroticism is reflected in the man who told us he felt his baby must be a girl because he so much wanted to please his wife during their lovemaking.

Accepting the pregnancy

The main issue of the first trimester, for men as well as for women, is to discover and accept the pregnancy. The woman is generally the first to suspect pregnancy, and generally the first to have her suspicions confirmed. In this age of sex education and sophisticated contraception, the man may be as aware as his partner is of a late period and may be with her when she takes a home pregnancy test. Perhaps he has even noticed that she has been slightly bloated, tired, or in other ways subtly changed. One man told us, "I thought she was pregnant. Her skin texture changed, something tactile that I picked up through my fingertips. I could never describe it." Nevertheless, men seem to find it hard to believe that these changes are related to pregnancy or the creation of a child. Even if they have seen the results of a home pregnancy test, men are likely to be skeptical. They seem to need a more authoritative statement from a doctor before they can "get" it.

A few women are secretive about "female matters." They may simply feel that men shouldn't be bothered about such things, or they may fear miscarriage and not want to share the knowledge until such a danger is past. Their partners may have to guess, or overhear whispered comments among the women, or finally notice a very enlarged abdomen and realize for themselves what is happening.

The way in which the father learns the news will probably be related to the way in which the mother expects him to react. She will know whether he has been eagerly awaiting a child or whether he dreads the possibility of having one. If she has been trying for years to supply her husband with an heir, she will tell the news in a very different way than if the family is already overburdened with many children.

A forty-year-old man will react differently from a sixteen-year-old; one who is in an economically sound position differently from one who is jobless and in debt. Some pregnancies will instantly bring joy, others anxiety. But the matter is hardly that simple. For each man and each pregnancy, there will be mixed emotions. Even those who dread making a woman pregnant may also feel tremendous pride in the proof of their masculinity implicit in fertility. Some cultures judge men by the number of children they engender rather than by any other display of talent.

There is a quality of selfishness about the flash of male pride that comes with making a woman pregnant. It may not fit with a more realistic picture of the father's role in family life. It may temporarily complicate the marital relationship, because it has implicit within it the idea that the woman is only a vessel for the man. Even wives with few leanings toward women's liberation may have trouble tolerating an attitude that accepts their own profound physical changes as a mere vehicle for someone else's achievement.

Some men are frightened by this glimpse of their own male pride. They may have been operating on the assumption of equality with their spouses, yet suddenly find themselves entering into a relationship that clearly delineates separate roles for each. But whatever the man feels, his wife will probably be seeking reassurance that he is pleased, that he will not reject her. She may not yet fully believe that she is pregnant, although she is getting some evidence from her body that it is true. The change has begun. Will the husband accept her when it becomes more marked? He has not yet had to face anything that affects him directly. She, therefore, may expect constant reassurance from him that he will still accept her and always love her.

From roots as deep and as primitive as these comes the

common fear of paternity—perhaps it is not his child? After all, there is no proof. This doubt, which can even nag men who have never before had reason to suspect their wives of infidelity, is probably based on doubts about their own masculinity. For a wife's pregnancy is the ultimate certification of a man's maleness. It is his contribution to society, and his link with immortality. With so much at stake, a man may wonder if he really could have been responsible for the almost miraculous event and its long-term consequences.

Shakespeare created a classic portrait of the psychotic father-to-be in *The Winter's Tale*. King Leontes falsely accuses his devoted wife, Hermione, of adultery with his best friend. To be a cuckold, that is, to be married to a woman who was having an affair with another man, was the ultimate humiliation in the Elizabethan era. The most terrifying possibility was that the husband might unknowingly raise another man's child. In his passion, Leontes tries to have his friend murdered and succeeds in having Hermione convicted of treason. When he finally comes to his senses, some time after the birth of a healthy daughter, his young son has died of grief, his wife is believed dead of shock, his lifelong friend is alienated, and his newborn daughter is thought dead of exposure at the king's command. Leontes seems to have converted his jealousy of the baby to a jealousy of his friend, to the destruction of all.

The relationship with the partner

The darkest fears of a pregnancy for the man are usually more than balanced by the miracle of the potential new life and the pleasure in new maturity. A husband may at first be pleased with the demands made upon him. His wife may seem to need more help and more love. She wants reassurance and, if morning sickness or tiredness shows up, he may feel proud to give a little domestic help, perhaps bring her breakfast in bed, or give her an understanding smile as she goes to sleep early. But if she is unable to get up *every* morning, or falls asleep *each* time he wants to make love, it is likely that he will lose his warm, protective feelings toward her and become more resentful and demanding. Perhaps he has just glimpsed the future.

At the end of the first trimester, the woman is entering the most regressed phase of her pregnancy. There is a profound turning inward toward fantasy. It is accompanied by a reassessment of her relationship with her own mother and an identification with the baby inside of her. She is not yet the baby's mother; she is part of it as it is part of her. In this identification with the baby, a wife may have strong and complex feelings about her own mother. Suddenly and irrepressibly, the wife is thinking, talking, and dreaming about her mother. She may phone her more often, praise her, condemn her, be almost obsessed with her. A husband may sense the intensity of his wife's involvement and feel that he is not the object of her concern. He may see a side of his wife's personality that he had not been aware of, or that he thought she'd outgrown. He may feel rejected and become resentful of his mother-in-law. A man may get his first taste of competition and envy at this time in the pregnancy. He may struggle to reach his wife through the cloudy haze in which she seems to be enveloped. If he fails to make contact, he may begin to feel disoriented and rejected.

Prenatal bonding

Early in pregnancy, a man has no positive evidence that he is gaining a child. In a normal pregnancy with no technological interventions, he can see only changes in his wife's body. "I had heard, 'When someone's pregnant there's a glow about her,' and said, 'Oh, sure.' But it's true. There's a fullness, as if all her cells are all ripe and full, and she has become this ripening person." The baby's heart may already be beating, but the father cannot yet hear it on his own, even by pressing his ear to his wife's abdomen.

If the expectant father gets to see a sonogram of his child-to-be in the first trimester, he will understand more concretely that his wife's changes are created by his child. This may be the first thing that makes it real for him. "I saw it moving around, these little hands and little feet. It's really a baby in there!"

Practical concerns

By the end of the first trimester, a sense of responsibility may begin to weigh upon an expectant father. He may reevaluate his job, his salary, his bank account, and his home. Insurance companies have learned how vulnerable the husband of a pregnant woman is and make a determined effort to sell him larger policies. A man may be surprised to find himself convinced by a sales pitch that never tempted him before. He may look for speculative ventures in the stock market. These financial issues are real, but they often get out of proportion to the actual needs of the family. They become the focus because they are something the man can be expected to handle. The activity may hide deeper worry about competence and security.

It is at this point that the expectant father searches for new pathways in his own life. He does not know that his partner will turn from her ruminations about her mother to ruminations about him. He knows only that she is retreating to a relationship that was dominant before he knew her. He may search for his own companions, who may also be a reflection of an earlier life-style.

The first trimester is a time when a man will begin to appreciate and experience those aspects of the pregnancy that are unique for him as a male, a father, and a husband. These experiences will be sex-linked, often unavailable to his partner and even antithetical to the supportive and affirming role that she may need and expect at this time. It is still too early for common issues of parenthood to unite them. If there is to be a mutual alliance during the pregnancy, it can be forged at this early stage, before the uniqueness of their experiences creates obstacles too great to be totally bridged. This alliance will require a peculiar blending of selfishness and understanding. It is all too easy to destroy the uniqueness of the experience for one of them because of the demands of the other. Too often, it is the husband who represses his feelings and needs, overwhelmed by his wife's more visible changes, especially in the first trimester when her only signs of pregnancy are likely to be nausea and fatigue, causing alienation where there could be a dynamic exchange.

A poignant reminder of the sacrifices demanded of an expectant father appeared in Herb Caen's column in the *San Francisco Chronicle* in December 1989; the item had been found in the classified ads of the *Sacramento Union:* "Motorcycles for sale: Honda 850, Odyssey 350. Mint condition. $1,750. Girlfriend pregnant."[16]

THE SECOND TRIMESTER

The relationship with the partner

Both husband and wife must remain open to the ecstatic and the awesome emotions of their partner. The differences in their experiences are part of their union. A woman may find it difficult to listen to her husband's fears about their financial future or to understand his unaccountable uneasiness about her rapidly enlarging breasts just when she wants to feel secure and attractive, but how else will she be able to find out what is really going on inside him? And how else will he be able really to listen to her own peculiar kinds of involvements? If they start to care about each other's anxieties, fantasies, and joys now, they will have an easier time following them later, and may even take pleasure in the inner growth of pregnancy.

Sexuality

Many of the physical symptoms of the first trimester will have abated in the second, but the physical changes of pregnancy are more apparent, especially for the multipara. The husband was not directly affected by nausea, fatigue, or indigestion, but he is dramatically affected by his wife's changing shape. Her breasts are enlarged and sometimes even secrete small amounts of thick milky fluid called colostrum. Her belly becomes increasingly distended, and her waistline gradually disappears. As Dan said of his wife in the fifth month of pregnancy, "Her breasts are bigger, her belly is filled out, she's really a woman. She's gone from like a violin to a cello, in a good sense, just full, the archetypal woman."

The most obvious effect these changes have is on the husband's sexual interest in his wife. A man may not be sexually attracted to a woman whose body is so different from the one he married. Verbal support and affection can be simulated, but sexual relations cannot. Unless the couple can talk about their sex life, their entire relationship may suffer, and that in turn will compound their sexual problems.

Sexual issues tend to become the focus in the middle trimester, when the visible changes begin. For many women, sexual excitement is at a new height. They become extremely passionate in a way that their husbands may not have encountered before. A passionate woman may be exciting, but she can also be very demanding—sometimes more than a partner wants to cope with, especially if he is unhappy with her changing body and unusual moodiness. Some couples reach new sexual heights during this phase of pregnancy; they convert a preoccupation with the growing baby and changing form into rich physical intimacy. This is a hidden plus in the pregnancy which can shape a couple's sexuality far beyond the child's birth.

Regression

The husband will find that his proximity to a pregnant woman can influence him profoundly. As we have remarked above, he may dream about changes in his own body, or about becoming pregnant himself. Forgotten childhood memories about his mother's or a relative's pregnancy may suddenly haunt him. He may feel intense envy and jealousy. Lying night after night with a woman whose body contains a living being may become frightening, particularly if there is already a strong basis for fear of women. The more that the husband identifies with his wife, the more intensely these emotions may affect him.

Almost all men have difficulty dealing with one or another of these very primitive emotions. Often, men cannot understand or cope with their own strong identification with the feminine aspects of their wives and particularly with the wish to be female themselves. The little boy who imagined himself to be pregnant was laughed at or ignored. This left a permanent legacy of hurt feelings which may be reexperienced around his wife's pregnancy. Positive residues about pregnancy may be even more difficult to deal with for men who are not sensitive to the feminine aspects of their psychological makeup.

There are no practical things to do to relieve the inner tension of the second trimester. Later on, the husband can involve himself in preparation for parenthood courses. But the second trimester has few such outlets. If a husband goes along on a visit to the obstetrician, he will see that the doctor *does* have a useful way to contribute to the pregnancy, and this may make him feel even more jealous and displaced. A few men become afraid as they realize that their partners may control all access to their child.

The woman usually remains in the inward and regressive state that began at the end of the first trimester, but her preoccupation tends to shift away from maternal figures toward people closer to her real world, particularly her husband. She may feel deep anxiety about his safety at this stage, and this sudden concern may make a man feel overprotected, as though his independence is being threatened. When a woman begins to make her transition toward motherhood, she becomes increasingly dependent on the husband as the major anchor of her new identity. She may become regressed in relation to him, expecting his help in things she ordinarily could handle alone, looking for approval and guidance in small household matters, and counting on him for decisions she previously made herself. Inevitably all her problems with authority figures will be projected onto him. She may become angry at any sign of weakness in him, or feel hurt and rejected if his attention wavers from her conversation. She may fear he will leave her, or she may be obsessed by a horror that he will be injured or killed. Some husbands learn to call at regular intervals rather than be interrupted unexpectedly by a distraught wife. A man who ignores his partner's anxieties may find they escalate rather than abate with a condescending "Everything is going to be all right, dear."

Prenatal bonding

If there has been no sonogram, the expectant father's first solid evidence that his partner is carrying a baby comes when he feels movement inside her abdomen. It plunges him into his coming fatherhood in an unequivocally physical way. He may first sense the tiny movements against his own body as his wife holds him tightly in bed. More commonly, he is asked innumerable times to touch her belly, and finally perceives the small bulges moving or discovers that when he pats a lump, it pats back.

For most men, feeling the child move against their hands is both exciting and disquieting. It brings to an end any lingering disbelief in the pregnancy. Larry, a professional artist, described the change in words of life-giving creativity:

> Since noticing movements, it's gone from an egg, sort of an amorphous blank that's getting bigger and bigger, to a fetus. At the sonogram, there was an instant that reinforced my calling it a he, where I was just sure it was a little boy. I saw a gestalt, just a form on the computer, but I thought, it's mine, it's mine!

The expectant father may spend a great deal of time touching the protruding limbs of the fetus, outlining its form, putting his hands on the woman's belly and waiting for the slightest movement. If he experiences the fetus in this physical way, he will, by proxy, be spending a great deal of time caressing his wife; acknowledging the growing child can become a husband's way of initiating lovemaking. Some men add scientific observation to their sensuality by carefully listening to the heartbeat or trying to imagine the anatomical part behind the bulge. The openness of the physical relationship between a couple will be an important variable in how the movements will be experienced.

It is hard to know how many men really take advantage of the opportunities to participate with their wives in these earliest movements. Descriptions of intense interest in the fetus sometimes come from men who seem conservative in their marital relationships. On the other hand, many men are embarrassed by such discussions, as though the subject were taboo. There are many ways of showing concern besides physical ones, but feeling the developing child in his wife's body will be the man's only way to put himself in touch with it until it is born. There is clinical evidence that a woman's mothering may be affected by her feelings about the moving fetus. There may also be a correlation between the way a father reacts to a child *in utero* and the way he treats it later.[17]

Fathers as well as mothers have pet names for the fetus and play with it by poking its lumps or singing to it. We interviewed an expectant father named Ray, who told us:

> I sort of flip-flop between thinking of Sarah as a single package and it being Sarah and "squink," which is our nickname for the baby. The first time I put my hand on her belly and felt the kid, it just changed it from being an inert, hard-boiled egg to being this critter. Here's Sarah, one being, but there's another life going on. Wow. Amazing.

There is a distinct advantage to being aware of stresses during the second trimester. It is a relatively quiet time, when the man's developing a few sympathetic symptoms that mimic the pregnancy in his wife won't get in the way of larger issues. A man can explore his more profound feelings about sexual identity and not be thrown off stride. If he indulges some of his slightly peculiar feelings, he may be less likely to find unexplainable or unanticipated emotions suddenly overwhelming him later.

THE THIRD TRIMESTER

By the end of the second trimester, the husband has begun to work through some of the psychological problems aroused by the pregnancy. The resurgence of primitive emotions such as envious and competitive feelings, the challenge of feminine aspects within his own personality, the responsibilities of prospective fatherhood, and the shifting relationship to his wife have each been confronted and dealt with. But those men who have sought ways to avoid the pregnancy experience will probably continue on that same path, throwing themselves into more work, taking longer trips away from home, developing individual or masculine hobbies, or becoming involved with other women. Only rarely will a particularly dramatic crisis—a near miscarriage or unexplained bleeding—shift this pattern. Some women who sense that they are losing their partners during pregnancy try frantically to involve them in natural childbirth or exercise classes. This alone rarely works. The psychological processes that prevented an earlier alliance are almost sure to be operative now.

Practical involvement

If a marital alliance has been forged, and if the man has been psychologically open to the pregnancy experience, the last trimester of pregnancy will bring rich insights and rewards. Unlike the first part of pregnancy, here the reality issues are in much sharper focus. A man can become involved in childbirth preparation with his wife, he can link her dependence on him to a critical event, and he can learn specific ways to take care of her that will have a real influence on her psychological and physical comfort. In this phase there are other ways to be directly involved in fathering. A husband may help his wife pick out a crib or carriage or design a nursery, or perhaps build a cradle. These activities are *for the child*, not for the wife, and may move a man forward in his inner sense of himself as a father. The financial issues he worried about before will be real now, as the medical expenses approach and as new housing requirements become essential. And as the baby's birth draws closer, he knows that he must prepare to take charge of the household while his wife is in the hospital or at home recovering from childbirth.

The relationship with the partner

The third trimester is a time when both husband and wife begin to emerge from their intense, separate inner worlds. The problems of the last trimester are the physical awkwardness of the woman, the potential medical difficulties of labor and delivery, and the imminence of the baby; they all require practical solutions. Up to this time, the challenge has been to accept and support the feelings of one another without much real sharing. Now, the anxieties are more concrete and understandable, and the need for working together is more obvious.

We interviewed a woman who was put on total bed rest because of premature labor. Her husband, who was working full time, waited on her hand and foot. We discussed the situation with him. Some might resent finding themselves in this position; Robert took pride in his active role. He was a good cook and prepared fabulous meals, including lunches which he stored in the freezer. Both partners felt they were involved in the job of making the baby twenty-four hours a day, and an arduous job it was, too, especially for him, but as he put it, "I feel as if my food is nurturing them both."

As the pregnancy moves toward its inevitable climax, the tension increases. Many couples experience a renewal of their relationship, a romantic bond that may have been missing over the past few months. If it is the first pregnancy, the coming of the baby may remind them that they will never be just a couple again. Their fundamental unit will change in an almost mystical way. As part of the added intensity of their relationship, a man may experience a new sense of tenderness and protectiveness toward his partner. She is awkward, and, by previous standards, unattractive. Yet she is at the height of her womanly potential, helpless, yet incredibly full and stirring with life. He may find himself taking care of her as if she were a fragile doll. He may carry packages for her, or take over her wifely and motherly chores. He can court her as he has not done since their first meetings.

Sexuality

There are very practical physical problems that the man must face if he expects to have sexual relations with his pregnant partner. By now it will be quite impossible to assume the same positions during lovemaking that they may have been used to. If the couple continues to have intercourse, there is a need for constant experimentation to decide, each week anew, what contortions are still possible and mutually pleasurable. Side-to-side positions or intercourse with the woman on top of the man are usually more practical during the last trimester, but a husband may be too embarrassed to attempt to experiment, especially at a time when his wife's body is so unfamiliar.

Some men and women may be frightened by their own interest and pleasure in sexual positions that were previously reserved for fantasy or for "blue" movies. On the other hand, the need for reconsidering sexual predilections may be long overdue for couples who assumed that their previous modes were adequate. A well-allied couple may find that the increasing anxiety of pregnancy may draw them together in ways that overcome minor sexual embarrassments.

Although obstetricians occasionally impose a limited prohibition on intercourse in the final weeks of pregnancy, some couples stop regular sexual contact long before that.

For one thing, it is a convenient excuse for bypassing the practical and emotional obstacles created by the pregnant anatomy. Some couples feel that the proximity of the penis may harm the child, or that the woman's orgasm may precipitate premature labor. Little objective evidence exists to justify these feelings, except when there is medical reason to be concerned about premature delivery. One couple who had delivered two babies prematurely stopped intercourse during the last trimester, waited till the nine-month gestation period was passed, made love vigorously, and brought on the labor contractions. Intercourse is also a folk remedy for poorly progressing labor. Many couples feel too restricted by the hospital environment to use genital or breast stimulation, but sometimes the staff encourages it by leaving the room after suggesting that the couple "get intimate." Intravenous drugs like Pitocin are the recourse of modern medicine.

Prenatal bonding

The reality of the coming baby increases each week. Body parts can be distinguished through the abdominal wall. The husband may now find himself dreaming of having a real relationship with his child. For example, most new fathers do not imagine the newborn, but see themselves walking with their two-year-old, or playing ball with a teenager. Fathers may wish fervently for a baby of a particular gender. One may want a girl to complement his family of boys, another a son to take after him. The closer the birth, the more reality-oriented these fantasies become. Special names and gender preferences may change dramatically for the husband as he focuses on the child already fully formed and almost visible through the taut skin of his wife's abdomen. Names that have seemed appropriate suddenly seem silly, adequate for something that was just a part of his wife, but not for a separate being that is as much his as hers. The two parents may suddenly realize that their notions of the child's identity are very different. The father may only really begin to understand his own ideas about fathering at this time in the pregnancy. Even an experienced father may find himself reevaluating these issues under the pressure of the unknown identity about to become real.

Prenatally, awareness of the baby is part of a new father's developing sense of himself as a parent and is more important as part of his identity formation than as actual behavior. His fantasies help him prepare for his future role. When we interviewed Ray, he said:

> I imagine myself changing diapers, no big deal. Yeah, it just threw up or pooped . . . it's a baby. Those are the things I expect. I want to see him begin to change. I imagine keeping an eye on him as he crawls around . . . watch it, he's getting into things over there . . . like that.

Preparation for childbirth

Anticipation is the overwhelming experience of the last month or two of pregnancy. The husband may realize that his wife is preoccupied with her womb in a new way. The "false contractions" that can begin as early as the sixth month now become increasingly relevant to him. He may feel beleaguered by his wife's requests to feel her contractions and to time them. He must reassure her that he knows how to get to the hospital, or that the money is available to pay the obstetrician. Although he cannot feel each contraction as she can, her anxiety can be contagious. Some men actually map the route to the hospital and make trial runs at various times during the day and night. Others become obsessed by the possibility of a flat tire or a malfunctioning ignition but how can he service the car if it might be needed that very night? He will have to keep in close telephone contact with his wife, and may be unable to concentrate at work.

A man can often become anxious about the possibility of a medical problem occurring either to his wife or to the child during the birth. Two of the husbands in the pregnancy study group were obsessed by medical danger and had nightmares about losing their wives in bloody catastrophes. Other men's dreams reflected their feelings of responsibility, that their wives might suffer because of what they had done to them. Some cultures and some women are particularly disposed to blame the man for impregnation, as though all sexuality were bestial and all of its consequences a painful burden imposed by the male.

Even if a husband does not actually feel guilty, he may be convinced that whatever happens is ultimately his responsibility. He must make sure that all of the arrangements have been made for a safe delivery. Because hospitals are thought of as places for the old and the ill, some men may be very afraid of delivery. They may never have been hospitalized themselves and know nothing about what they may regard as the mysteries of medicine. A few obstetricians seem to emphasize the dangers of childbirth, as though to enhance their own role and the skill it requires—all further increasing the father's anxiety.

THE BIRTH

Since childbirth is the culmination of pregnancy, it seems appropriate that the pregnancy experience should end as it began, in an intimate, shared moment between a man and a woman who are creating a new life together. Convention used to dictate that the father be excluded from the delivery room. In some hospitals, he was not even permitted into the labor room. The American husband had to sit out the long hours of labor in a dreary waiting room, to be told of the birth by a nurse or an aide who was a total stranger. Then he might be allowed to see his wife briefly and get a glimpse of his new baby through the glass partition of the nursery. He and other family members were separated from the new mother, except for brief moments, for almost a week.

Earlier this century, George Bernard Shaw caustically described the typical birth:

> When the terrible moment of birth arrives, its supreme importance and its superhuman efforts and peril, in which the father has no part, dwarf him into insignificance: he slinks out of the way of the humblest petticoat, happy if he be poor enough to be pushed out of the house to outface his ignominy by drunken rejoicing. But when the crisis is over he takes his revenge, swaggering as the breadwinner, and speaking of Woman's "sphere" with condescension, even with chivalry, as if the kitchen and the nursery were less important than the office in the city. [18]

Shaw was describing the male role in an old-fashioned home birth. Comedian Bob Newhart updated the description for mid-twentieth-century American men in the hospital waiting room: "You're the lowest form of life. Even maintenance men will have nothing to do with you." [19] Many men were not unhappy to be excluded from the childbirth experience. They were willing to deliver their wives into the competent hands of a modern obstetrical staff. In the sixties, even when hospitals allowed husbands to coach their wives, many chose not to participate.

Men seemed reluctant to attend births for the same reasons that they felt estranged from the entire pregnancy experience. As Shaw suggested, childbirth is the ultimate feminine secret. It symbolizes the mystery of creation. There are cultures that say that a man would die if he saw his wife in childbirth. American men used to have an informal humor that approached a mythos of fear around childbirth. Men were thought unable to manage a birth even in the case of an emergency—with the notable exceptions of doctors and fabled New York City cabdrivers. Hospitals seriously opposed the movement toward allowing men into the hospital by claiming that they would faint or otherwise disturb the doctor. There was almost no rationale for such beliefs. With very little preparation, men have proven quite capable of contributing to rather than hindering a woman's experience with childbirth.

Sometimes, a woman does not want her husband around while she is giving birth. She might feel embarrassed or insecure in his presence, or she may feel that it is not in his realm—and she may be right. This position is expressed in an extreme form by a Japanese legend:

> Long ago an empress was observed by her husband to turn into a dragon during labor. She was so mortified when she realized he had seen her that she fled, leaving her child behind.[20]

Many women in our culture are afraid that they will do something embarrassing or inappropriate during labor, perhaps a fear based on the behavior of women in previous generations who gave birth under the influence of "twilight sleep."

If a husband has not involved himself in the pregnancy, there is little reason for him to be expected to change at the last minute. Other people become the support and resource for this event: mother, sister, friend, midwife, or physician. The husband may not fit in. Perhaps his job was to get his wife to the hospital and pay her bill. Among the men in the study group, Brenda's husband, Bob, chose that role.

He had full access to the labor room, but he chose to spend most of his time in the waiting room. He helped his wife by bringing her a soda from time to time and by keeping in telephone contact with his mother-in-law. He was inept at more intimate contact and could not see when she was too involved in labor to respond to him. He tried to get her attention while she was in the middle of a hard contraction and put his hand on her shoulder when she would not answer him. This was extremely difficult for her; she was happier with him out of the room and preferred to depend on the doctor and on medication for relief from discomfort.

Some men are disturbed by the intensity of their partner's labor contractions and afraid of seeing blood and the surgical aspects of childbirth. That is understandable. It is difficult to see someone you love struggle to deal with pain. There are problems with the protector role: a man can't protect his wife from the experience of birth; she must go through it. He may mediate the experience by encouraging her, but if he is overprotective, he will not be a help. A labor coach is a guide more than a guardian.

In the actual event, as in the fearful anticipation of the third trimester, the trip to the hospital becomes a convenient focus for fear and anxiety that most men feel, and it often becomes a symbol of their sense of incompetence and helplessness in the face of forces over which they have had no control. Movies and television comedies typically show a frantic husband driving at dangerously high speeds on the trip to the hospital, racing down wrong-way streets, chased by a policeman on motorcycle, who joins in as an escort, and then pulling up, exhausted, at the wrong hospital! If men cannot negotiate the distance between their homes and the hospital without such blunders, how can they be expected to behave responsibly in the fragile sterility of the hospital delivery suite? Most of the old stories were apocryphal; even before childbirth preparation classes, men were able to understand what was going on. But we did know a man who carefully waited until his wife's contractions were four minutes apart, then left with her for the hospital but could not be dissuaded from picking up a hitchhiker whom he drove ten miles out of the way despite his wife's groans and complaints. Another man stopped with his wife to watch the sunset on their way to the hospital, then backed into another car on his way out of the vista parking lot. Regardless of how much preparation and sophistication a man may have, the ride to the hospital becomes a focus of responsibility and tension.

The husband's role in childbirth has been revolutionized since 1970. Now most hospitals *expect* the partner or some other support person to accompany a woman in labor and to be with her while she is giving birth, unless there are complications that require surgical intervention.

What of the experience of the man who has been allowed to participate actively in the birth of his child? Can he escape all the anxiety, fear, and boredom that are so much a part of the nonparticipating husband's experience? Probably not. Labor is long and arduous work. It is also a lonely, solitary time. No matter how involved the husband may become, he cannot perform the work of dilation and of expulsion of the infant. He is a servant to the needs of his wife and interpreter of her wishes to the hospital staff. He is closer to the action, but that also means that he is closer to experiencing the primary pain and fear of a critical event. At best, his role is that of supporter and comforter, helping her believe that she *can* do it.

Most contemporary hospitals are staffed with people who are used to dealing with partners in the maternity unit. They know how to explain their rules and how to help a man feel welcome. Nevertheless, the father-to-be may feel angry and uncomfortable at his treatment sometimes. He is an outsider in hospital territory. He may feel relegated to an unobtrusive corner—or he may feel that they are leaving too much up to him. What does he really know, not having been through this before? Well-trained, sensitive nurses on family-centered maternity units will recognize his dilemma and help him gain confidence.

Laboring women often complain of experiencing the hospital as cold and hostile. Husbands, too, can develop a paranoid perception of the sterile halls and officious staff. If a man wants to create a warm, protective sphere within which his wife can labor in confidence, he must overcome both fear and anger. He must find a middle path. If he is skillful, he can draw extra attention and cooperation from the staff; if he is careless, he can alienate them and create a hostile environment. If he must leave his wife's side for some reason, he should know that she is with people who like her, who understand what she is doing, and who will try to help her. Husbands who argue with the doctor about a routine examination or who refuse to allow their wives medication when they obviously require it may make things worse for everyone, including their wives, even when they are trying desperately to be helpful.

One of the most frequent complaints from physicians is that well-intentioned partners simply do not understand the time involved in a normal labor and become distressed with their wife's discomfort. They push for relief before the woman asks for it. The staff may feel that they have two patients on their hands. The complaint from fathers is that they are shoved aside by the obstetrical team instead of being treated with respect and concern.

Martin Greenberg, a psychiatrist who has written about his experience at his son's birth in his book *The Birth of a Father*, described his feelings about the use of a fetal monitor during his wife's labor:

> He then plugged her up to a machine.
> Let me tell you what I mean by that. He reached up into

the birth canal and placed electrodes on the baby's head. He explained that the monitoring equipment would provide a continuous check on how the baby was doing during labor . . .

It seemed as if the machine had taken over. In fact, it was now physically located where I had been sitting . . .[21]

As a physician, Martin Greenberg was familiar with hospitals and unintimidated by medical procedures, but still he felt displaced and disoriented by the machinery.

A husband has an important place at his wife's side. During the long stretches in which there is no staff person in attendance, he will be a companion for her. During difficult moments of examination or medication, he can be a real support. At first, he may feel embarrassed to use the breathing routines he learned in preparation classes. He may hesitate to move a pillow or in any way disrupt hospital property without specific permission. But he will begin to feel more at home as he realizes that he is performing a more and more necessary service for his wife during each contraction. His voice is a comfort to her. He will see her need for him. It will not all be easy for him. She may turn to him during a contraction, looking with frightened eyes into his face, as though he were the only thing she had to hang on to. He may feel her begin to grow tense and want to shriek with fear himself, but instead he says the calming words that he memorized in practice sessions. He will see each of the recurrent gushes of water or blood and realize that the sequence of events is not as simple in real life as it sounded in the books or classes. Feeling that the life of his entire family is on the line, he may have to listen to the casual banter of nurses while they examine his wife, or watch the frown on the doctor's face as he comes to check the progress of dilation. Minute by minute, with little to look at but the slowly moving hands of the clock, he hears his wife's breathing going through the progressively more difficult phases described in preparation classes. He must try to guess how she feels about proffered medication and even make the decision for her when she does not seem to know whether she should take something or not. As he wipes the sweat from her brow, he may feel that he is in the middle of the worst experience of his life and tremble at the awesomeness of its outcome.

Some people question whether or not the father is the best coach during labor. He can't ever have gone through it himself and may be feeling guilty for making her suffer, since it is he who made her pregnant. He may be nervous and uncomfortable in the hospital, anxious to keep his partner from feeling any discomfort and, in a conventionally masculine way, need to *act* in a situation that calls for patience and trust of nature. There is no universal answer to such a question. Some laboring women want to depend on another woman, someone who has been through it herself. Many cultures exclude men from births and use the woman's mother or, occasionally, her daughters as her assistants. For many American families, the father is an ideal choice. For many others, he finds a more comfortable role as companion but has an experienced person take on the role of coach.

The climax of his experience will almost certainly occur when he hears the baby has crowned and is about to emerge from the birth canal. If he is in a hospital that uses a full delivery room, he may be overwhelmed by the display of medical technology. He may feel out of his element, without any practical function whatsoever. But precisely because he has no technical function, he can experience the event for what it is, an important moment in his own life.

A new father may have a more exhilarating experience at the birth than the woman. He is under no physical distress and often has a clearer view of the infant. Sometimes, especially in the case of a cesarean section, the father may be the first one to hold and get to know the baby, may be the one to hand it to the mother.

Fathers frequently describe the awesome moment in which they first confront their newborn with as much enthusiasm or more as mothers do. Perhaps it is the more intense because it is often unexpected. Martin Greenberg calls this "engrossment," which he defines as

> a father's sense of absorption, preoccupation, and interest in his baby. He feels gripped and held by this feeling. He has an intense desire to look at his baby, to touch and hold him. It is as if he is hooked, drawn to his newborn child by some involuntary force over which he has no control. He doesn't will it to happen, it just does. Often he has this experience when he sees his baby for the first time, and especially if he participates in the birth of his child.[22]

Occasionally, a husband is brought to childbirth preparation classes against his will. But a reluctant man should try the classes; many get hooked when they start to learn more about the experience. If his reluctance to participate is based on problems in his relationship with his wife, however, the skills he acquires in childbirth classes will be too superficial to compensate for the lack of trust already present. His training may even work against the laboring woman, for his presence can introduce tension, keeping her worried about something other than the event at hand, and deflect the attention that the hospital staff might otherwise give her. The stresses of labor and delivery are too profound to support a foundering marriage. Former tensions are more likely to be exaggerated than reduced by the intimacy of the process.

When a couple is motivated by a sincere desire to share in every aspect of the experience of pregnancy and childbirth, the husband's involvement will enhance the alliance that has already been formed. They will see their relationship in a new light, and enter a new phase of life together.

6

The Fourth Trimester

THE EARLY WEEKS

OVER AND OVER AGAIN women and men say, "Why didn't anybody tell me it was going to be like this?" Caregivers (doctors, nurses, childbirth educators, therapists, and even grandparents) reply, "We tried to prepare them; why didn't they listen to what we were saying?"

Something about the postpartum period is ineffable, inexplicable, unprecedented in life experience. One can't know in advance what it is going to be like because it consists of more than the facts. The postpartum experience includes profound inner changes that sweep over the couple just when they both need to develop a whole new set of practical behaviors. The baby needs to be taken care of; the mother needs to recover from childbirth, learn how to take care of a baby, and learn to feel good about herself as a mother; the father needs to learn how to take care of his recovering wife, learn how to take care of a baby, and learn to feel good about himself as a father. A baby *needs* everything; what about a new mother and a new father? Who takes care of their needs?

Physical recovery

Pregnancy may technically be over at birth, but in reality, the physical changes linger postpartum. For a woman, the early weeks are dominated by the birth experience, by the strangeness and vulnerability of the baby, and by regaining the balance of her body, which does not return to its pre-pregnant state instantly.

Many women have to recover from surgery after child-birth. They may have had either a cesarean section (major abdominal surgery) or an episiotomy (a minor incision in the perineum). Either one requires stitches and hurts until it heals. Even without stitches, a woman may be sore from the events of birth: the stretching, the descent of the baby, the manipulations by the medical attendants. The uterus typically takes weeks to return to normal. The *lochia*, or bleeding, continues for several weeks and is a reminder that the new mother's body is still recovering. Less visible but equally important, a woman may still be trying to under-stand and master her sense of the events of the birth. She may be able to attend to little else as she replays the events blow by blow. She will benefit from having someone who was there that she can talk with.

A breast-feeding mother's breasts may be sore and her nipples cracked; for many women, the first three weeks of breast-feeding are acutely uncomfortable. Even if she adores her infant and wants very much to breast-feed, the woman's pain can affect her mood and make her feel inadequate. If she does not know it will pass, she may give up and feel like a failure. Consultation with a lactation expert can help, for these feelings sometimes have an unfortunate (though temporary) influence on the mother-child relationship. As one new mother told us, "I was a terrible grouch in the first two weeks. Every time the baby latched ahold of my nipples, I just stiffened up with the pain. Thank goodness he was my second baby. I knew it wasn't always like that, and sure enough, it improved with time."

Sexuality

Some women want to have their partners caress and love their bodies when they are vulnerable and sore. Kissing and fondling may feel relaxing and healing. Most are too tender to find touch to the breasts or genitals comfortable. In the past, the couple may have taken care of each other's sexual needs even when one was not feeling very erotic. This kind of sexual play becomes a difficult burden for a new mother. She is spending so much of her time and energy taking care of the baby and using her body to serve its needs that she may begin to wonder whether her own breasts belong to her or not. Sexual requests start to feel like demands; "You, too?" she may ask when he wants to make love. She is not feeling his love; she is perceiving his need, and she is re-acting from her own need to protect herself from feeling used. He is expressing his need to be loved, too. It hurts him to be excluded from the mother-child cocoon.

The baby

For both the new father and the new mother, the baby finally becomes "really real." Babies are famous for crying and for waking in the night. These two attributes may make them much more difficult to live with than one can imagine in advance. There are quiet babies that cry seldom and comfort easily. Even so, the baby's cry is a reminder of its helplessness. Someone must be finely attuned to every aspect of an infant's being. That someone is usually the new mother; her attention is always directed toward the infant, sensing its rhythms, anticipating its cries, perhaps more aware of its needs than her own or, of course, than her partner's. If she does take her mind off the infant for a few moments (whether to make love or read a novel), it seems to have an uncanny awareness of the change and screams for her renewed attention. She is so attuned to the baby and the baby is so attuned to her, but she cannot always comfort it. Sometimes, no matter what she does, she feels inadequate. No matter how much preparation she did, no matter how hard she tries, she cannot be a perfect mother.

In the first weeks after childbirth, the mother and the baby are still united in a symbiotic bond. Psychoanalyst D. W. Winnicott refers to "primary maternal preoccupation,"[1] his name for the psychological state typical of new mothers as they are absorbed with their infants. It is as though an invisible emotional umbilical cord still links the two together. A new mother describes her experience:

> That I responded to him as quickly and thoroughly as I did, that his call roused me as urgently as it did, was surely a form of love. It simply wasn't a type of love with which I was acquainted. This was love on a cellular, biological level. Intimacy, I began to understand, is rooted in the corporal. It has to do with the distance between bodies. None separated mine from my son's. We had both been swallowed by the cave I used to fashion for myself under the covers, that safe, familiar space which traps the odors of your own body— milk, blood, tears, sweat all mingling. This wasn't the romantic intimacy between adults, but an earthbound, often tedious kind which is undertaken, no questions asked.[2]

Babies evoke much more complicated feelings than can be imagined. Even experienced parents can find themselves surprised by the reality of caring for their new child.

The new mother's emotional needs

Every baby needs to be close to a comforting body, and the mother is biologically equipped to offer hers. But mothers are people with needs of their own; sometimes they need to get away from their babies. For many women, unbroken contact with their children is anxiety-arousing as well as exhausting.

A woman may find herself in the midst of a personal reevaluation after the baby is born. Bonnie was a thirty-two-year-old woman who had just given birth to her second child. Her first was born eight years earlier with a young and irresponsible man. Bonnie had spent most of the early years with her first child as a single mother in a rural area. Then she married Brad, a man who lived in the suburban community in which he had been born and raised. Her in-laws and neighbors all took a concerned interest in her well-being. A few hours after her second daughter was born, Bonnie took a painkiller and went to sleep. She woke up in the middle of a nightmare in which a terrible crime was taking place right next to her. For the next two weeks, she found herself preoccupied with her past, going over the details of her wild "hippie" youth in excruciating detail. She felt unworthy of her husband, who was serving her gourmet meals in bed and was thrilled with their new daughter. She was embarrassed at being so nasty and withdrawn in the face of such generous love. When Brad cheerfully picked up the baby and carried her with him to the kitchen while he tidied up, Bonnie was overwhelmed with feelings of inadequacy and even suspected that he was just doing that to show her up.

Then Bonnie started thinking of her grandmother, the most consistent and loving figure from her childhood. And Brad continued to tell her that she was not being as much of a grump on the outside as she was feeling on the inside.

He marveled at her ability to tolerate the discomfort of her perineum. He praised her for her ability to soothe and caress the baby even when she cringed with pain when it sucked on her nipples. She and Brad vowed they would never separate, no matter what. He told her he wanted to grow old and grouchy with her. Bonnie felt accepted and loved in a way that she had never experienced before. She realized that she was grateful to be living the life that she had held in such contempt fifteen years before—the life of a suburban wife and mother. Her period of withdrawal was a period of mourning for her old life and a coming to terms with the reality of her new life.

Many women feel that they give up more than they gain, at least in the short run. Bonnie, in contrast, felt that she had gained more than she deserved. As she recognized, hers was a "lucky" problem. The next six months became the happiest period of her life.

Many women get "the baby blues." We don't mean the hormonal roller coaster of the first week postpartum period or the desperate depression of a woman who stops functioning in the months after she has had a baby. We are referring to the irritability, fatigue, difficulty concentrating, and low self-esteem that come over formerly active, sociable women who suddenly find themselves alone at home with a baby. The new father may be her primary or only support person. Does she have anyone else that cares what she is experiencing from day to day, with whom she can discuss the confusing little mysteries of infants? How many other people know how inadequate she feels sometimes? She may need her partner more as a friend, confidant, and "mother's helper" than as a lover. She will need someone to validate her experience. In our culture, young parents often lack a supportive group to help them understand their new role in life and must fall back on each other for help.

A woman's partner is the most important source of support

for most new mothers. Researchers have discovered that the best way to predict depression in a woman after childbirth is to measure the mood of the father in the middle of the pregnancy. When he is depressed during the pregnancy, she is much more likely to become depressed postpartum.[3]

Confinement

Our society used to talk about the period around childbirth as "confinement." The term itself conjures up images of imprisonment, restriction, and deprivation. One is "confined" to bed when one is sick. Does that mean new motherhood is an illness? Are childbearing women taboo, that they should be confined to quarters?

For all of the negative associations that we may have with the term confinement, the actuality of bed rest and restriction from usual activities is extremely important for a new mother. Only the poorest societies do without what Shakespeare referred to as the "childbed privilege." Slave women had no choice but to work immediately after childbirth. Similarly, peasants around the world, like the one in Pearl Buck's novel *The Good Earth*, must pick up their newborn and return to the fields.

We Americans, who so value the workplace and the outside world and frequently denigrate the importance of domestic work, often yearn to return to "normal" activities as soon as possible. We isolate our new mothers instead of creating a position of honor and comfort for them.

Many cultures provide for the physical and emotional readjustments of the new mother. They honor parenting and nurture a new mother much as they expect the mother to nurture her child. Anthropologist Soheir Morsy reports that Egyptian peasants see "confinement" as an indication of their valued status. They are given the time off because they have done something so important in their society, not because they are taboo.[4] In China (Taiwan) it is called "doing the month"; the new mother stays home for a month and is free from all of her usual responsibilities.[5] In rural Japan, a woman must wait one week before performing any household tasks, three weeks before doing strenuous work.[6] According to an anthropological study, one group of Chinese peasants makes sure that new mothers get chicken to eat every day for the forty days of their ritual after-birth period. This is a great privilege in a society that rarely affords the luxury of meat.[7]

We have no ritual markers to define the postpartum period, so it is hard to say how long it lasts. Physical recovery may occur quickly after an easy birth. Most women find a gradual resumption of physical strength and a gradual interest in resuming normal activities. The quality of their experience depends on how the people around them react.

The meaning of motherhood

The way a woman incorporates parenthood into her life may surprise an outside observer. For example, a teenager who finds pregnancy stressful and at odds with her expected place in society may have a relatively easy postpartum adjustment.

Sally, a seventeen-year-old high school student, married her boyfriend and continued to attend school. Her pregnancy was extremely uncomfortable. She felt "everyone" (especially her parents) now knew about her sex life. She cried much of the time and felt terribly embarrassed in the corridors of her school.

As soon as the baby was born, Sally found life delightful. She and her husband lived with her parents. Her mother did most of the housework and helped with the baby. A neighbor cared for the infant when Sally returned to school.

The baby itself was like a living doll to Sally. She loved playing with it, bathing it, and feeding it.

While Sally found pregnancy a nightmare, she found motherhood a joy. Everyone around her was helpful and she was amazed to discover that she was a good mother. She grew into the role gradually. She did not lose much of her old life; she simply gained a new baby. She wasn't ready for all the responsibilities of running a household, supporting a family economically, or nurturing many children, but that was not what was needed from her. She had time to mature into her role.

Jane was a thirty-two-year-old school counselor when she decided that she was "ready" for motherhood. She had waited four years after marrying because she wanted to make sure that she and her husband "had time to get to know one another" and to be financially secure. When she felt secure, she stopped using contraceptives and became pregnant within four months.

Jane adored being pregnant. She felt special, alive, and radiant. She continued to work and felt that everyone was envious of her condition. She had not lost anything, but had gained a special treat.

Postpartum, Jane took a nosedive. Suddenly, she was overwhelmed. When the baby cried, she could not always make it stop. Her husband worked long hours and became irritable when the baby fussed through the evening. Her friends from work stopped dropping by. She felt lonely and incompetent and yet was overwhelmed with guilt every time she thought about leaving the baby to return to a job that she felt she knew how to do.

Jane's parents were far away; her husband and her friends did not know much (or care much) about baby care; she was lonely and bored. Worst of all, she found that she was not the perfect mother she had planned to be. Her expectations of herself were so high they could not possibly be met. She, like many women her age, was caught between her desire to be a good mother and her desire to continue her career with minimal disruption. Sally had felt none of these conflicts, for she had not had her life disrupted.

Work

Most women take at least a few months' maternity leave. The early weeks may be free of the immediate stress of work, but the issue of return is sure to receive attention. Some women look forward to getting back to a familiar role. They are secure in their work identity and receive self-esteem from their performance on the job. Parenting does not provide such clear rewards. Many women dread the need to return to work and feel that they are going to be torn away from their most important role when they leave their baby with a sitter. Most new mothers are concerned about fatigue. How will they find the strength to go to work every day *and* take care of the baby at night? Women must face these questions as they are learning to care for their babies.

The new father's feelings

Now that men are encouraged to be involved in pregnancy and to be present at the birth, wonderful things are happening. New fathers get to hold the baby and fall in love with it. Many of them take paternity leave to get used to the new family situation and to adjust to their new roles. With these expectations, however, come disappointments for new fathers that parallel those of new mothers.

Men get little validation of their parental experience; they are expected to devote themselves to taking care of their wife and providing for the family. A man hopes to feel like a father and instead he may find he is handmaiden to his wife.[8]

Perhaps the hardest feeling for a new father to deal with is his jealousy for the baby, who always demands and gets his partner's attention—and her body. What could be worse than a two-week-old rival? If he succeeds in establishing as close a relationship with the baby as his partner has, he risks evoking her jealousy. Now that there are three, someone always seems left out.

The new father may have an important role taking up the slack with older sibling(s) after the new baby is born. The mother is recuperating and preoccupied with the infant. Occasionally, the reverse occurs. The mother may be unable or unwilling to separate from her older child. The new baby may become the father's; he then becomes the primary caregiver.

Most men find that they cannot stay in a close relationship to the new baby unless the mother encourages them. If the mother is breast-feeding, she has that extra, intimate contact with the baby and has a built-in way to comfort it. She is usually with the baby more hours than he is. So much of the infant's waking time is dedicated to feeding and changing. If the woman has to do the feeding, the father is left with the changing, a distant second.

Pamela Jordan, a researcher at the University of Washington, discovered that

> men in this investigation wanted to be involved parents, but they did not believe they had the knowledge, skills, or support to do so. They felt alone in their experience and without resources to enact the parental role as they ideally would have chosen. Their motivation was impressive. Viewing the experience of expectant and new fatherhood through their eyes provided insight into the myriad of obstacles impeding their role enactment. Data indicated not malicious or purposeful exclusion, but benign societal neglect. Despite a general perception of blurring of gender roles in our society,

the delineation of parental role expectations is still along very traditional lines.[9]

In the beginning, the father may be relieved to return to work, to a job that he knows. In a few weeks, he will get an important boost when the baby starts to smile and show recognition, squeal with delight when he comes home from work. He will feel important.

The early months are frustrating for a man who yearns for closeness. Jerry, a writer who took care of the baby every morning while his wife, Jane, worked, struggled for recognition in his nurturant role. Jane believed that Jerry was irritated by the baby's disruptions of his work and resentful of taking care of the baby. Jerry said:

> It has its frustrations, depending on the stage of my writing. I was used to working in an absolutely quiet environment and I don't have that anymore. But I am adapting. They are just new demands, that's all.

Jane perceived him as more resentful than he seemed; she also told us that "he's a man and they like children when they are older, not when they are younger and messy." Her own beliefs about men and infants kept her from being able to recognize or appreciate the nurturant behavior of her own husband.

Fathers often become the more playful parent. We have heard breast-feeding mothers complain, "He can comfort the baby without feeding it. Whenever I hold her, she wants to nurse!"

Much of modern society still makes traditional assumptions about men and women, mothers and fathers. Formal psychology discusses the role of the mother and the role of the father based on such assumptions. We should remember that both Freud and Jung were raised as nineteenth-century

Europeans. They saw the father as the separator, the one who first comes between mother and baby, who leads the child out of the symbiotic attachment to seek life outside the nursery. But that is not all a father can be. Instead of helping by symbolizing the outside world, he can help by willingly valuing the "inside" world of the home, of nurturance, and of child care.

We feel it is best for both parents to become adept at comforting the baby and playing with it. All three will benefit from a warm and effective relationship. The new father may not have breast milk, but that means that the baby will get used to other forms of care from him. He may find that he becomes better at distracting the baby and comforting it without resorting to food. Creative families can find solutions for the discrepancy between the maternal and paternal experience. The new father can carry his infant in a Snugli on walks; he can take it on a ritual trip to the bakery on Sunday morning; he can be the one to give the baby its bath. These special moments create a routine of involvement that assure the father of a real role inside the family.

The couple's relationship

Women who enter parenthood with the expectation of equal involvement feel betrayed and abandoned as they take on more and more of their former life. Ann was a creative, energetic, competent, and hardworking businesswoman who also happened to be tall, graceful, and well dressed. When we met her, she was the mother of a three-month-old baby conceived and carried to term after four years of infertility.

Ann said that she had been pleased at conception; it proved her femininity and womanhood after they had been in doubt. But she said she had become increasingly distressed as pregnancy progressed. She had even considered an abortion but was talked out of it. She stopped all sexual relations in the fourth month.

After the baby was born, Ann felt rage at

> everyone who told me I could do it, who said things would get better in a little while. They said that mother-love would just come; well, it hasn't. I've tried to take the baby to work with me, but then I can't talk to my clients. I have a baby sitter, but some days she doesn't make it. My husband would never miss a day of work to stay with the baby. Why should I? And when am I going to do the shopping for the dinner party we are having Saturday night? I haven't even sent out the thank you notes for shower gifts, much less Christmas cards. Everybody seems to expect me to be energetic and excited. I just feel exhausted and depressed.

Kathy had eagerly looked forward to motherhood and enjoyed pregnancy and the first postpartum month—until her husband, Ken, accepted a raise when the baby was six weeks old. Ken started traveling a lot and Kathy was haunted by dreams in which she was separated from Ken. When Ken was away, Kathy found she could not comfort the baby when he cried. She just held him and rocked and cried and rocked and cried.

Many women feel abandoned by husbands who promised they'd help out. They feel invalidated—as though child care was not important enough for their husbands to do, and certainly not as important as the money they could earn in the workplace. If staying home with the baby is such a privilege, why is no one there with them?

Marion's situation was like Kathy's. When her husband, Marty, became involved in an extra project at work and stayed away long hours, she started thinking about returning to teaching. Ironically, now that Marty was working such long hours, he was adamant that Marion should be staying at home with the baby. He did not want anyone else doing it. She wanted to be more like him, to move more freely outside the home.

BEYOND THE EARLY WEEKS

When does the postpartum period end? This is not a simple question. We have called this chapter "The Fourth Trimester," implying that the postpartum adjustment lasts three months. In fact, most families have established something of a routine by the time the baby is three months old. The woman's body is more or less stabilized; the baby has something of a routine going. But when we look at issues of parental identity, few families have reached a point of stability by the end of the third month. Reva Rubin states clearly, "It takes nine months from childbirth for a woman to feel like herself again: whole, intact, functional."[10] Nine months is a good estimate for a woman who is the primary caregiver for her child. But even this does not acknowledge the pervasive sense of connection that parents, and especially involved mothers, feel toward their children.

Physical recovery

Beyond the early weeks of recovery from birth, breast-feeding women experience ongoing changes, especially in their genitals. They have a hormonal profile that is close to that of menopausal women: a reduced supply of estrogen makes their vaginal walls thin and slow to lubricate. While a new mother may be too dry down below, she is often too wet up above. Lactating breasts often leak when a woman is sexually aroused.

Sexuality

One marker of recovery from childbirth and return to other aspects of normal adult life is the return of a sexual relationship between the new parents. Most couples go at least a month after childbirth before trying to have sexual intercourse together. Many find that they do not feel ready until long after that. We've talked with men who've waited four to six months. Occasionally, a couple has not renewed their sex lives a year after their baby was born. This sometimes happens because they tried once or twice but it did not go well and they were afraid to try again.

A breast-feeding woman can enjoy sex, but, for largely physiological reasons, she will probably find that it takes her longer than usual to get aroused. She may also be afraid of getting pregnant again, because she knows that she would not be strong enough to do a good job with a second child so soon after the first.

A new mother may not seem very interested in getting started, or if she agrees to try, she may not respond to lovemaking in the same way that she used to. The new father must remember that he has not lost his touch as a lover; his wife simply has a higher threshold of arousal. To get results, both partners will have to be more motivated than in the past. A new father will also discover that her body feels different. Her belly is soft, perhaps even flabby, and her breasts are large and full. Her vagina, too, is mysteriously changed.

Most of us agree that sex is for more than conceiving children. Sexual contact expresses love, hate, caring, aggression. Sexual excitement can be play, delight, or frustration. Sexual release can be satisfaction, comfort, ecstasy, or terror. In a loving couple, sexual intercourse is an expression of emotional unity and a dynamic exchange of giving and receiving pleasure. Sex is a way of taking care of someone;

it is also a way to feel taken care of. Why does this become a problem in the postpartum period? Part of the reason is that the woman may not yet have conceptualized herself as a sexual being *and* a mother. The two roles are often kept separate in the minds of both men and women.

Many Americans say that women use sex to get love and men use love to get sex. We have known many men *and* women who experience sex as proof of love and feel rejected, even devastated, if their partner does not want them sexually.

A new mother sometimes gets nervous when she is starting to enjoy herself. She may feel that if she sinks into selfish pleasure, she is abandoning or betraying her baby. She wants to put the baby's needs before her own pleasure. She may feel guilty about having fun and feeling sexy and may not yet have learned that parents have to take good care of themselves in order to be relaxed and happy with their kids. Children flourish under the care of a father and mother who love each other and who give pleasure to each other.

The couple's relationship

New parents are really in a new relationship. They have to woo each other all over again, like new lovers. Perhaps intercourse isn't the way to start. They must reexplore each other's bodies. Hers is not the same. She may not know how to anticipate her own responses. He may feel estranged from the new breasts and changed vagina. They are like a couple of adolescents exploring new territory. Warmth, closeness, and open communication are more important than intercourse or orgasms at first. That will only follow if the couple feels secure and loving with each other. When the baby is well enough established in the world, it is time for the new parents to work on their own relationship.

Work

Another important marker for a new mother's return to normal adult life is her relationship to the outside world. When she resumes household chores and shopping, she is fully functioning, though she may still feel groggy and unlike herself because of lack of sleep. When the baby's rhythm of eating and sleeping is predictable enough for her to get regular periods of rest, she will feel more able to be effective in other areas of her life. This may include going back to a job outside the home, but it may also involve other areas such as community involvement, full-time domestic responsibilities, or creative work.

Whenever we have joked with an audience of parents that the postpartum period lasts at least fifteen years, we have heard an enthusiastic "yes" in support of our statement. As long as children are dependent on their parents, those parents find themselves preoccupied with thoughts of their children. This does not keep them from enjoying other aspects of their lives, but it does mean that they never return to being quite the same people they were before they were parents.

7

Conclusion: Six Psychological Tasks of the Childbearing Year

PREGNANCY IS a relatively short developmental stage that inaugurates a much longer one: parenthood. As a period of transition, the childbearing year can be used to get ready for the complex and challenging tasks ahead. Deep and meaningful feelings must be recognized and respected. Men and women work at becoming parents not just by learning breathing exercises and changing diapers, but also by facing feelings from the past, exploring insecurities, looking at fears, and accepting strengths and weaknesses.

Over the years, we have seen that parenthood develops gradually. Parents in their second and third pregnancies seem eager to work on psychological problems that they did not deal with the first time around. They have learned how important it is to confront issues that affect parenting. It is an ongoing process, not a time-limited event.

The six psychological tasks of pregnancy explored in this chapter have all been discussed implicitly and explicitly in earlier chapters. They are presented here by way of summary, rather than to introduce new concepts. Each task should be explored as it emerges, to resolve rather than ignore the issues, for new tasks arise and the expectant parents must be ready to confront new challenges as they come along.

Parenting draws on all aspects of ourselves, both on the external level of nurturant behavior and on the internal level of identity and selfhood. The childbearing year can be used to achieve new levels of personal strength and clarity of purpose.

Task #1: To accept the pregnancy

The first task is to recognize the pregnancy, then to accept its reality and do something about it.[1] Sometimes the choice is to terminate the pregnancy in abortion. In that case, there are no expectant parents; the other psychological tasks do not have to emerge (but the fact of the abortion will come up later, when the woman chooses to carry a pregnancy to term).

Pregnancy may be denied or misinterpreted if the emotional need to do so is great enough. Every emergency room nurse seems to have at least one story of a teenage woman who arrived at the hospital with intense abdominal cramps that proved to be labor contractions. The baby arrives as a surprise, not only to the woman herself, but also to her family. No provisions have been made. One wonders about the quality of care the infant will receive—and the quality of relationships in the life of the mother.

A woman whose mother had trouble in pregnancy may have a superstitious terror of following in her tracks, compounded by a fear of succeeding where she failed. For example, Sonja had felt detached from her long-planned pregnancy. Suddenly, in the middle of the second trimester, she was overwhelmed with a memory of a horrible second-trimester miscarriage her own mother had had when she was four. She could remember the bright red blood on the white bathroom tiles. Sonja realized why she had been so detached from her own pregnancy. She breathed a sigh of relief and relaxed into her own experience.

Refusal to accept the reality of the pregnancy is an unhealthy form of denial, for pregnancies have consequences. They do not just evaporate; when they are over, there is a baby to deal with. Only by accepting that reality will a woman take proper care of her health and begin the process of appropriate parenting. Even if the baby is to be given up for adoption, the pregnant woman must acknowledge her condition to ensure that the baby will be cared for—and that she herself will receive good medical and emotional support.

Men generally lag behind women in believing the pregnancy is real. They do not miss a period, feel tenderness in their breasts, or become queasy at the smell of coffee. They often have to wait for stronger evidence—diagnosis from a doctor, a sonogram, a bulge, or fetal movement— to believe it is real. Thus men may have a shorter period of psychological gestation for their parental identity. This may be all right if they do not have to make any radical changes to accommodate for the child, but it can be difficult if there are extreme adjustments to be made.

For some people, pregnancy is more an end in itself than a means to an end. For a woman, it may fill an inner void, make her feel creative, productive, and full of life. Similarly, men may feel inspired by a pregnant woman as a symbol of the life force. The abstractions may be so enthralling that there is no realistic preparation for a baby, for the end of the pregnancy. These men and women stay fixed in Task #1.

Task #2: To accept the reality of the fetus

Babies gradually become more and more real to the parents. Some people have a distinct image of the baby even before the pregnancy. They are already "in love" with their child and experience a spiritual connection with it. In such cases, failure to conceive or failure to carry the pregnancy are particularly distressing. For women who have strong fantasy images of their babies, the unsettling symptoms of pregnancy can be a healthy reminder that the unexpected can happen, and that it is important to accept the child as he or she truly is and not project rigid expectations onto him or her. One woman who was three months pregnant said in a support group: "I felt more like I was going to have a baby two months ago, at the beginning of the pregnancy. Now I just feel pregnant." She was absorbed by fatigue and nausea, by being pregnant, not by having a baby.

Parenting is a continual accommodation between expectations and reality, between the parents' projections about who they think the child is and the child's own nature. It is healthy for this accommodation to begin early. The dreams and anxieties about the fetus that are so common during pregnancy may be a creative part of this process, which is so like the imaginative play of childhood. Particularly for women, doll play may have been a precursor of the relationship with the fantasy child that is so present in the second half of pregnancy.

In the first trimester, pregnancy often seems to be only a change in the woman's body. This is true symbiosis. Psychologically, the expectant mother cannot and need not relate to the baby as anything other than a part of herself. As evidence of independent life emerges, the symbiosis will give way to the beginnings of a real relationship with reciprocal needs, a process of incorporating this child as part of the self and developing a parental identity that is specific to this child.

Nancy, a member of a support group we led in the eighties, craved bagels during her pregnancy. When she told her husband, he said, "If the baby wants bagels, she'll get bagels." (He knew the baby was a girl from prenatal testing.) Nancy immediately thought, What about *me!* Then she had another thought. Maybe she wasn't being ignored. "He is parenting the child in me," she said. She felt herself—that symbolic, childish part of herself—and the real fetus taken care of simultaneously. The bagels couldn't be for the fetus without also being for Nancy. In pregnancy, they are wrapped up together. The couple can practice the complicated levels of need and nurturance that must be addressed after the baby is born. When the father said "for the baby," the mother was at first jealous and then reinterpreted his remark to mean "the baby in me" and so felt nurtured herself. The father was ahead of her in separating pregnancy from fetus, mother from child.

A sonogram can increase the reality of the baby and facilitate attachment (prenatal bonding). It can also bring fantasies and a sense of the baby as part of one's own body to a sudden halt. Parents often feel a rush of love and attachment and are more ready to receive the baby into the family after they have seen it on the screen. As one father said:

> It might not have been so powerful if it had been a high gloss photo of an embryo, but since there were sort of gaps and I had to fill in, there was something of a mosaic image, and I just saw it. That's my kid! It's something where your awareness is expanded. You had that flash. It was automatic.

At mid-pregnancy, this combination of projection and reality is stage-appropriate. Viewing the sonogram images may loosen the symbiotic state characterized by a woman's inability to distinguish the baby's needs from her own needs and encourages the perception of the woman and baby as separate.

While the sonogram encourages perception of mother and baby as separate, it need not foreclose fantasy. For example, Nadine, a dark-haired Italian woman with a dark-haired, dark-eyed husband, who knew her baby to be a girl, continued to see a blue-eyed boy in her fantasies. She was aware of two processes going on simultaneously. On the one hand, she was choosing a name for her little girl, and on the other, she was imagining herself as mother of a baby boy. The two images came together after the birth, when the real mother, Nadine, held the real baby, Sarah.

Both the sense of union and the sense of separation are important to parenting. In pregnancy, both parents can fantasize about the baby and play with the idea of connection, with an image of the baby as part of themselves, and also play with the idea of it as a formed individual. The real personality will not begin to interfere with the fantasy for a few more months, and even after the baby is born, its personality will emerge gradually.

Task #3: To reevaluate the older generation of parents

The next issue to come up in pregnancy is the confrontation with the "other" parents, sometimes still experienced as the "real" parents, the mother and father from one's family of origin. During the middle of pregnancy, while the fetus is becoming real and being conceptualized as a baby, it is natural to look to other fathers and mothers, to see who they are and how they performed as nurturers.

Characteristically, it is late in the third month or early in the fourth month of pregnancy that women become absorbed in the process of reevaluating their relationships with their mothers. The reevaluation seems to happen whether a woman expects it or not. She finds herself dreaming about her mother, increasing the number of phone calls and/or visits per month, and in other ways showing symptoms of a renewed interest in her. Women also find themselves thinking about their fathers in different ways, especially in ways that compare their fathers with their husbands. Women in a support group in the eighties expressed concern that their husbands not feel alienated from the family, the way their own fathers had. As one of them said, "My father was happy when we kids left home because he finally had his wife back to himself!"

To reject one's mother without seeing her as a whole person viewed with compassion often activates a similar rejection of the mother in oneself, because women identify so profoundly across generations. We saw this most dramatically in a woman we will call Jennifer, who came to psychotherapy because she was six months pregnant and suicidal. She said that she had a loving husband and had wanted to have a baby. At first the pregnancy was fine, but then she became anxious, apparently for no reason. Thoughts of death overwhelmed her; she was full of schemes for killing herself.

We quickly learned that Jennifer rejected her mother in childhood and had based her adult adjustment on trying to be the antithesis of her mother. That had worked well for her until she felt the baby move inside her womb and she realized that she was going to become a mother. She literally decided that it would be better to kill herself, the mother in her, than to risk becoming like her own mother.

Jennifer's conflict had been unconscious. As soon as she articulated it, the anxiety diminished and she was able to realize that underneath the rejection of her mother there was another layer of feeling, a layer of profound attachment. She still did not approve of her mother, but she found that she could become aware of both positive and negative feelings and be accepting both of her mother's fallibility and, fortunately, of her own fallibility as well. This is an important part of the task: to develop compassion for the inadequacy of parents in preparation for the inevitable failures and disappointments that will also occur in the new family.

The feelings of love, hate, frustration, satisfaction, dependency, and rebellion that are a part of every parent-child relationship will never be more relevant than during pregnancy. The hopes and expectations for each additional child bring new revelations about the problems and potential inherent in the mother-child relationship. The hope is to accept those qualities of the mother that were respected and valued and cast out the more negative, unwanted identifications while developing empathy for and acceptance of someone for who she really is, flaws and all.

A career woman is especially likely to identify with her father. Pregnancy entails a shift from being like him to realizing that she is entering a role he cannot model. Even if he was the more nurturant and loving parent and is the model for "mothering" behavior, he has no uterus, no breasts. When she is pregnant, she cannot reflect her own body image off memories of his body. But his approval for her uniquely female function is extremely important. Dotty dealt with this issue in her unconscious by dreaming during pregnancy that her father came to her dressed in her mother's nightgown and robe. Her mother had died when Dotty was little; her father had been the only available parent in her memory. She used him as both mother and father.

Men engage in a similar process, though it may start later in the pregnancy. They, perhaps even more urgently and with less satisfaction than women, look to the world around them for validation and, too often, find little support for involvement on an intensely personal level as a nurturant parent. The fathers of the current generation of parents typically played the role of breadwinner and were excluded from intimate interactions, especially with infants. Like the fantasies about the baby, the search for good models is part of the evolution of parental identity within the self.

Jack came to psychotherapy after separating from his pregnant wife. The main topic in his therapy became his father, a powerful man who had in many ways been the primary parent when his mother became too sick to take care of him. "Why does he always find the flaw in everything I do?" Jack complained. "Why can't he ever praise me?" Jack did not want to become such a figure for his own child. When Jack returned to his wife, he continued to be confrontational and competitive with his father, but he created a very different style with his son. He found himself drawn to his favorite uncle, an unsuccessful but warm man. He also paid close attention to the ways women handled babies. After he had clarified his feelings about his own father, Jack was free to turn to alternative figures and learn from them.

Part of the process of reevaluating the relationship with parents is to realize that they are no longer responsible for taking care of the family; that burden has shifted to the new generation.

Task #4: To reevaluate the relationship between partners

Both men and women often feel increasingly dependent during the middle of pregnancy. One must realize that he or she will not be taken care of by one's parents and that one's partner is not just a romantic figure but a life partner, a person who will shape the nature of the family system that will grow in importance over the next two decades and more.

This may be the first time in the marriage that dependency issues have been important. Suddenly, women wonder if their husbands will take care of them. They test them through bizarre requests for such things as pickles and ice cream. Men wonder if they will be abandoned when their wives are busy with the new baby. They often have dreams of being locked out of the house or shut out of a room. Feelings of desertion are disconcertingly common during pregnancy. Can you turn to your spouse, even with your irrational needs? Will he or she take care of you? Can *you* take care of him or her? Are the two of you mature enough to be entrusted with a fragile infant's life?

An important study of expectant and new fathers showed

> the mother is in a key role to bring her mate into the spotlight or keep him in the wings. The most promoting mothers seemed to share the fathers' view that gestation, parturition, and lactation were privileges rather than burdens. These mothers brought their mates into the experience by frequently and openly sharing their physical sensations and emotional responses. They also actively encouraged their mates to share the experience of becoming and being a father . . . The truly sharing mothers were few.[2]

The new mother is important to the father's experience; reciprocally, the new father is critical to the mother's experience. Studies of mood through pregnancy and the postpartum period have shown that if the expectant father is depressed during the pregnancy, the new mother is likely to become depressed postpartum.[3] His mood, his feelings about becoming a parent and having a baby, affect her experience. Especially if she will be home alone taking care of the baby, he stands between her and isolation. If he does not value what she is doing, it is extremely important she find other sources of validation (support groups, therapy, family, friends). If she does not value what he is doing, he will feel left out and estranged. Women ask: "Will he be there for me?" Men ask: "Will she let me in?"

The partner is the front line of validation and support for struggling with new roles, for finding the meaning of parenthood in relation to self-esteem. This is not true in all cultures. When men and women live in distinctly separate worlds, they receive support and esteem from others of their own sex. Many men and, especially, women in America also feel more intimate with friends and relatives of their own sex than with their partner. For them, Task #4 entails reevaluating the relationship with that important group.

Phil and Tina, a couple who had always felt that it was "the two of us against the world," found that pregnancy changed their assumptions. When Tina, who had been estranged from her mother for eight years, suddenly reestablished contact, Phil felt betrayed. Even worse, he became afraid Tina would become like her mother. His main feeling was of abandonment. He was unable to conceptualize the dyad becoming a triad. Instead, he felt only rivalry, having come from a family that used the strategy of "divide and conquer." He, like all new parents, needed to create a new three-way relationship as well as to reestablish the marital relationship in a new way—as parents. For some, divorce seems easier than sharing.

John and Lindsay, a couple who had always wanted to have children and to enjoy family life, saw it another way. John said, "When you know you're going to have a baby together, it's like the relationship goes from black and white to color. This is the fulfillment; this is what makes a marriage real."

The husband and wife face the pregnancy together. Each one is part of the other's turmoil of the present and hope for the future. Each requires something from the other at a time when it is particularly difficult to give. The couple needs an expanded marriage relationship, a new alliance. This alliance cannot simply be a series of financial discussions or a joint decision to move to a new house, a new neighborhood, or a new school district. It is, most of all, an emotional alliance, an agreement to be sensitive to one another's needs, to communicate what is needed *now* from one another, to share experiences, to help the other cope with the unfamiliar and frightening events. It must be an alliance to allow growth in each individual and in the couple, growth enough to support the infant they both will care for in the future. It is their new *parental* alliance. Even if they choose to divorce, to discontinue their personal and marital alliance, they will have to continue to communicate around parenting issues and share decisions in the best interests of the child.[4]

Task #5: To accept the baby as a separate person

Toward the end of the pregnancy, most people are anxious about the birth. Couples are tired of the pregnancy and ready to greet the baby in the outside world, but they may also be sad to "lose" the pregnancy. In the ninth month, women may feel nostalgia for the special period of waiting, the time when dreams of the future are as important as action in the present. The baby will not be as easy to care for when it can cry and mess diapers and needs to be fed.

If the emotional investment was in pregnancy rather than in the baby, or if the *idea* of being a parent is abstract and idealistic rather than practical and real, Task #5 may cause trouble. Some parents do not want the baby to exist as a separate person who insists on being heard on its own terms; they are more content with a fetus who (in fantasy) floats contentedly within the womb. Others are eager to honor the individuality of the baby. Dan, who felt misunderstood by his own father, found the idea of parenthood challenging. He said:

> As the pregnancy goes on, I get more and more evidence of this upcoming baby. I think a lot more about being a father. I want to be able to both be identified and close to this baby and also to be able to see the person on his own and realize he has his integrity, his life all by himself.

There is continuity from pregnancy through the post-partum period, from fetus to newborn. By the time the fetus is developed enough to have a semblance of consciousness, the womb is already getting cramped. The fetus no longer has the freewheeling room to toss and tumble that is apparent in first- or second-trimester sonograms. After it is born, a nine-pound baby from the womb of a first-time mother wants to be swaddled tightly, for he is used to a secure fit on all sides. A six-pounder who spent his or her prenatal time in a well-stretched womb may move his swaddled arms restlessly, unused to being tightly bound. Parents often conceptualize a magic child that is a projection of perfection rather than a real infant that cries and squirms and throws up. After it is born, the mother will see a characteristic movement and recognize a sensation from pregnancy, crying out, "Oh, that's what it was!"

The moment of physical separation is the birth itself. Birth is a complicated psychosomatic event that is generally ruled by the physiological process. The psychological work or labor is the work of pushing the baby from the inside to the outside, of separating. *Postpartum* literally means "after the separation."

Bonding, the intense attachment that occurs between parent and child in the first hours or days after birth, is parallel to the feeling of merger that occurs during pregnancy. Bonding is an expression of empathy and connectedness, but it is no longer a connectedness with a fantasy child. The real child is there to be explored, encountered, reacted to. Bonding entails sensitivity to the child's needs, not the imposition of the parent's needs on the child. While the first few hours after birth may be a particularly open and intense time for parent-infant attachment to occur, the feelings of wonder, discovery, bemusement, and connectedness are part of the complex, lifelong love relationship that is the basis of a parent's ability to nurture her or his child. Some new parents feel their love come in a sudden flood; most find that it grows slowly over time. It is based both on the fantasies already developed and on the reality to be discovered.

If the baby dies, is given up for adoption, or is born premature, sick, or deformed, Task #5, to accept the baby as a separate person, becomes extremely difficult and perhaps even more important to explore. Parents must accept the reality of the child to which they gave birth and give up the fantasy of the child they expected. When a dramatic problem presents itself right away, the new parents must go through a sudden accommodation rather than gradually discover the reality of *this* child over the years of parenting. A new parent who never gets to know her baby because it dies or is taken away from her does not get to work on these issues in relationship to the child. She may feel as though a part of herself has been amputated and have no way to comprehend the feelings of incompletion and confusion that she experiences. In the past decade, our society has taken great strides toward helping parents understand their loss through support groups and counseling.[5]

In psychotherapy, a new mother invariably brings her baby to therapy with her immediately after the birth. At some point she decides to leave him or her at home. This natural separation occurs when the new mother is comfortable with other caregivers, but it is also influenced by the evolution of needs. Immediately after childbirth, the needs of the mother and the needs of the infant are compatible. As the mother of a three-year-old told us recently, "I did not expect early motherhood to be so *animal*. The baby was this little critter and I was its mother. Our connection continued to be almost as physical as it had been during pregnancy." Over time, however, the needs of the mother and the needs of the child change. Mothers want to think and talk about their own issues. A six-month-old becomes too distracting in therapy. Even when it is "good," that is, when it is happily curious about its environment and engaging others in relaxed play, a baby keeps its mother from accomplishing certain other goals.

During pregnancy, merger was simply an acceptance of two organisms functioning as one. When the infant is born, mother and child are still finely attuned and physiologically interconnected, especially during breast-feeding. Gradually, they separate and become interested in different activities. This is true for both of them. The mother (or father if he becomes the primary caregiver) may find herself with a renewed interest in hobbies or with a desire to return to her old job after weeks, months, or years. The baby will find that eating and sleeping and being taken care of by Mom are not enough anymore. The infant will stare in fascination at its fists or kick its legs with devoted energy, discovering its own power to influence the universe. Both parent and child are discovering (or rediscovering) the world beyond their dyad.

Some people parent from an aloof position, some from a merged position. Task #5 is the process of discovering one's own preferred level of connectedness and adjusting it in relation to the needs of other family members.

The progression from acceptance of the pregnancy to an awareness of the fetus to an attachment to the baby is one of increasing separateness as the individuality of the infant increases, but the separateness is still a relative thing. Babies need to remain psychologically merged for many years. They are not born able to function socially on their own. Good parents develop the ability to connect as much or as little as the child requires at each stage and to be sensitive to sudden spurts of independence as well as regression into total (but temporary) connectedness.

When the baby's separateness is experienced, the parents

must confront their own separateness and rediscover who they are as parents and as individuals.

Task #6: To integrate the parental identity

Parents have their own needs for merger, some appropriate, some inappropriate. For example, a mother may want to hold her baby because she needs comfort at the moment. This may work out occasionally, but sooner or later the child will feel the parental attention as an imposition.

The image of Madonna and child is a favorite because it evokes a sense of comfort in us all. The great artists are much less likely to capture the moment that follows the beatific vision, the moment when the pudgy six-month-old begins to turn his or her head from the breast and to squirm to get out of Mommy's confining arms. If, at this moment, Mommy still needs the comfort and security of the Madonna image, she is going to find herself confused by her sense of abandonment, and the child may begin to feel it has to take care of its mother by remaining a dependent infant. Parents have to learn to stay connected, but from a strong, empathic position, not from a needy, merged position.

Every new parent wants to feel good about herself in her new role, but if she has a difficult or colicky baby, she will have a harder time integrating parenthood as a positive part of her sense of herself. The child's temperament and its fit with the parent's is an important factor in the parent's developing sense of her own identity.

As the baby develops into its own, separate person and is not a visible part of the mother's body, the mother is no longer as totally enveloped in childbearing. Someone on the street might not know she is a mother. She may look much as she did the year before, but in fact she does have an important new role in her life. How does she integrate this with her ongoing sense of herself? Sometimes it is hard for a new parent to remember who she was in her old life. Some new parents are happy to let go of the old self. Many hunger to rediscover it. In her book about pregnancy and the first year of parenthood, Roberta Israeloff writes:

> Sleep when the baby sleeps, everyone always told me, in a tempting, rockabye voice. But how could I sleep away the only moments I was free to be myself—that is, connected with the person I used to be?[6]

The baby cannot survive on its own, but that is not the same as saying the mother must be totally devoted to it all the time; parents need to take responsibility that some loving and appropriate person is always with it, but it need not be themselves.

Many women are afraid of being trapped in traditional female roles, especially if they have developed an adult lifestyle that does not include nurturance or domesticity. For them, full-time motherhood may make it especially difficult to feel like "themselves." Their work identity may serve as a stabilizing influence in the face of dilemmas posed by pregnancy and early infant care. Here, at least, a mother may feel competent and comfortable while she grows into her new sense of herself. As one mother said:

> Coming back to work was almost like starting a new job. I was a different person. Now I was Amanda's mommy. At the office I am starting to feel like myself again. I'm getting to be myself and Amanda's mommy, both.

Pregnancy creates a new life for the parents as well as for the infant, but eventually they wonder what happened to their old life and yearn for things to be as they were before. The mother and father will want to be alone with each other and alone with herself or himself sometimes. The time comes when each must assess how deeply he or she has changed. Has she taken on a whole new identity, a whole new life-style, or just added a few new roles to the old self?

Some people feel that parenthood is discontinuous with their earlier identity, but others don't feel they have changed much at all. For some, parenthood is the fulfillment of the life that he or she always expected. The degree of disruption is related to actual changes and to the meaning of the changes. If someone else is providing full-time care for the new infant, the changes may not be as great. But there is almost always significant inner change. Even the most uninvolved husbands, who feel rejected and alienated from wife and child, know that they are now fathers. If there is no change to correspond to that knowledge, the person is alienated from a part of himself.

Change is stressful even when it is healthy and happy. The meaning of the change depends on the interpretation of the individual. What is the meaning of being a mother? For many women, it is associated with suffering and martyrdom. For example, Barbara's mother died of breast cancer when Barbara was just entering puberty. In Barbara's unconscious, mature womanhood was associated with pain, suffering, and death. She was able to enjoy life as an adult, but when she became a mother, she unconsciously assumed that she had to give up "fun." She could not grasp the concept of being a happy mother. Fortunately, Barbara had married an unusually playful man. He was strongly attached to the girlish side of her and was determined to keep it alive and active. Gradually, Barbara found that she could bring together her old, playful self with her new, responsible self. As the baby grew older and able to giggle and play, it became easier and easier for her to let go of her old images and learn to be a joyous mother.

Not all men reach the developmental stage of integrating a truly new identity with parenthood. They may choose to stay with the identity of wage earner and provider and not become involved fathers, not take on the behavior of a nurturant parent who is attuned to the nonverbal needs of the infant. In her study of new fathers, nurse researcher Pamela Jordan concludes:

> It necessitates great commitment and perseverance on their part to stay with the task of involved parenting. Many who reach it cannot maintain the effort. The ability to enact the role of involved father is strongly influenced by the supporting or nonsupporting environment created by the recognition providers. The rewards of involved fatherhood seemed worth the effort.[7]

The work of pregnancy is ongoing. A man in therapy during his wife's second pregnancy had a dream at the beginning of the third trimester that eloquently expressed the process for him. Sam had been talking about his own father and his envy of his wife, Polly, who was an effective parent and had been able to keep her career alive, suspending it for six months when the first child was born, then continuing part-time. She was planning to resume full-time work when the second child was a year old. Sam was dissatisfied with his job as a building contractor, but even more important, he yearned for greater acceptance in his family. Then he had this dream:

> Polly was going to a group meeting with other women. I left her there and went to a job site, which turned out to be an underground house that was being built by many people, young and old. It was a real community effort. I realized that they were building this house for me. I was very moved.

When he woke up, Sam realized that he had been receiving support for his parenting role from friends and from coworkers. When he thought of the people who were in his dream, he realized with sorrow that his own father was not among them. He was sad to give up hope for ever gaining positive regard from his father, but happy to realize how many other people were helping him build a very special life. Sam constructed his paternal role with the help of many people, young and old.

Like marriage or death, pregnancy is one of life's great rites of passage. It is a time of transition between one identity and another for both of the parents. Perceptions of the outside world, of relationships, of one's own body, of one's self-image shift during the childbearing year. Dreams and fantasies are more insistent and revealing. Memories, long buried and forgotten, suddenly come to light. All this psychic stirring creates an opportunity to explore the length and breadth of one's personality and identity, one's conscious and unconscious being.

The overriding psychological task of pregnancy is to integrate experiences from the past with the demands of the present. This emotional preparation for parenthood may be as important as the physical preparation for childbirth. Facing the issues may create emotional conflict or discomfort for a while, but the process of resolving or alleviating the conflict is important for developing the ability to be a good parent.

There is rarely a conflict between the emotional well-being of the fetus/infant and the psychological development of the expectant parents. They are almost always linked. Severe anxiety and depression are more likely to result from *not* dealing with fears and frustration as they come up in the pregnancy, and they are more manageable during this time than they may be after the child is born. The more problems are ignored or denied, the greater their influence. Ambivalence is normal; when it is suppressed or denied, it generates tension and anxiety.

*   *   *

Our division into six separate tasks clarifies the experience of the childbearing year, but we must remember that it is an artificial construct. In their normal sequence, the evolving awareness of the pregnancy, the fetus, and the child stimulate the development of the parental identity, including a reevaluation of the parental figures and a reevaluation of the relationship with the partner, as well as evoking practical nurturant behaviors. The tasks overlap and blend with each other when they are lived out in the lives of real people.

Those parents who are able to explore the meaning of each of the psychological tasks and achieve some satisfactory resolution to the personal problems raised by them cope best with the new roles and changing relationships of childbearing.

Notes

Prologue

1. See Arthur D. Colman, "Psychological State during First Pregnancy," *American Journal of Orthopsychiatry* 39 (1960): 788–97, and "Psychology of a First Baby Group," *International Journal of Group Psychotherapy* 21 (1971): 74–83.
2. Arthur D. Colman, M.D., and Libby Lee Colman, Ph.D., *Pregnancy: The Psychological Experience* (New York: The Seabury Press, 1971).

1 The Meaning of Pregnancy

1. Maxine Margolis, *Mothers and Such: Views of American Women and Why They Changed* (Berkeley: University of California Press, 1984), 47.
2. Ibid.
3. Steven Mintz and Susan Kellogg, *Domestic Revolutions: A Social History of American Family Life* (New York: The Free Press, Macmillan, 1988), 178.
4. Christopher Lasch, *The Culture of Narcissism: American Life in an Age of Diminishing Expectations* (New York: Warner Books, 1979).

5. Boston Women's Health Collective, *Our Bodies, Ourselves* (New York: Simon and Schuster, 1971).
6. Bruno Bettelheim, *A Good Enough Parent: A Book on Child-Rearing* (New York: Vintage Books, 1988).
7. Alexander Eliot et al., *Myths* (New York: McGraw-Hill Book Company, 1976), 216.

2 The Expectant Mother's Experience

1. Professionals and lay people alike are sometimes offended by the use of the word "crisis" in relation to pregnancy. The term is being used not to mean "trauma," as it often connotes in daily usage, but rather to mean "turning point" or "trans-formation," a period of greater susceptibility to distress. See Gerald Caplan, "Psychological Aspects of Maternity Care," *American Journal of Public Health* 47 (1954): 25–31.
2. J. Parks, "Emotional Reactions to Pregnancy," *American Journal of Obstetrics and Gynecology* 62 (1951): 339.
3. S. M. Tobin, "Emotional Depression during Pregnancy," *Obstetrics and Gynecology* 10 (1957): 677.
4. Ibid.
5. S. Saltzman and T. Schneidman, "Psychological Study of the Woman." *A Demonstration Project in Prenatal and Early Postnatal Adaptation, Final Report* (Washington, D.C.: U.S. Department of Health, 1968), 7.
6. Jellemieke C. Hees-Stauthamer, *The First Pregnancy: An Integrating Principle in Female Psychology* (Ann Arbor: UMI Research Press, 1985), 25.
7. A. J. Rosenberg and E. Silver, "The Psychiatrist and Therapeutic Abortion," *California Medicine* 102 (1965): 407–11.
8. I. W. Gabrielson et al., "Attempted Suicide Among Pregnant Teenagers," *American Journal of Public Health* 60 (1968): 2289–2301.
9. Daphne Maurer and Charles Maurer, *The World of the Newborn* (New York: Basic Books, 1988), 20.
10. For a provocative overview of fetal consciousness, see Thomas Verny, M.D., and John Kelly, *The Secret Life of the Unborn Child* (New York: Summit Books, 1981). For a more scientific

update, see Daphne Maurer and Charles Maurer, *The World of the Newborn*.

11. Nancy Sharts Engel, "An American Experience of Pregnancy and Childbirth in Japan," *Birth* 16 (1989): 83.

12. Hilde Bruch, *Eating Disorders: Obesity, Anorexia Nervosa and the Person Within* (New York: Basic Books, 1973), 276–77.

13. Andrew Lang, ed., "Rapunzel," in *The Red Fairy Book* (New York: Dover Publications, 1966), 282.

14. Ibid.

15. For a longer look at the dreams of pregnancy, see Eileen Stukane, *The Dream Worlds of Pregnancy* (New York: Quill, 1985).

16. R. D. Gillman, "The Dreams of Pregnant Women and Maternal Adaptation," *American Journal of Orthopsychiatry* 38 (1968): 688–92.

17. Ibid., 690.

18. Ibid.

3 The Stages of Pregnancy

1. Infertility is a large issue beyond the scope of this book. For a discussion that includes the psychological and social impact, see Barbara Eck Menning, *Infertility* (Englewood Cliffs, New Jersey: Prentice-Hall, 1977).

2. Elizabeth Hall, "When Does Life Begin: A Conversation with Clifford Grobstein," *Psychology Today*, September 1989, 43.

3. For a clear and complete discussion of prenatal testing, see Robin J. R. Blatt, *Prenatal Tests: What They Are, Their Benefits and Risks, and How to Decide Whether to Have Them or Not* (New York: Vintage Books, 1988).

4. Hall, "When Does Life Begin," 44.

5. For a probing discussion of the emotional issues related to abortion, see Sue Nathanson, *Soul Crisis* (New York: New American Library, 1989).

6. See Susan Borg and Judith Lasker, *When Pregnancy Fails* (New York: Bantam, 1988).

7. See Elisabeth Bing and Libby Colman, *Making Love During*

Pregnancy (New York: The Noonday Press, Farrar, Straus and Giroux, 1989).

8. William H. Masters and Virginia E. Johnson, *Human Sexual Response* (Boston: Little, Brown and Company, 1966).

9. Helen Wessel, *Natural Childbirth and the Christian Family* (New York: Harper & Row, 1963), 73.

10. Barbara Katz Rothman, *The Tentative Pregnancy: Prenatal Diagnosis and the Future of Motherhood* (New York: Viking, 1986), 104.

11. Ibid., 129.

12. Gale Lee Bernstein and Yasue Aoki Kidd, "Childbearing in Japan," in *Anthropology of Human Birth*, ed. Margarita Artschwager Kay (Philadelphia: F. A. Davis Company, 1982), 105.

13. Hees-Stauthamer, *The First Pregnancy*, 95.

14. Masters and Johnson, *Human Sexual Response*, 153–56.

15. See Bing and Colman, *Making Love During Pregnancy*.

4 Birth

1. Brigitte Jordan, *Birth in Four Cultures: A Crosscultural Investigation of Childbirth in Yucatan, Holland, Sweden and the United States* (Montreal: Eden Press Women's Publications, 1978), 74.

2. Ibid., 36.

3. Walter Radcliffe, *Milestones in Midwifery* (Bristol, England: Wright, 1967), 18.

4. For a critique of the factors thought to influence the cesarean rate as well as evidence that the rate of increase is slowing, see Helen I. Mariesking, "Cesarean Section in the United States: Has It Changed Since 1979?" *Birth* 16 (December 1989): 196–202.

5. See Bonnie Sullivan, *The Cesarean Childbirth Experience: A Practical and Reassuring Guide for Partners and Professionals* (Boston: Beacon Press, 1986).

6. Our focus is more on the psychology of pregnancy than on birth itself. There are many excellent books that focus on childbirth in greater detail. See, for example, Penny Simkin,

Janet Whalley, and Ann Keppler, *Pregnancy, Childbirth and the Newborn: A Complete Guide for Expectant Parents* (New York: Meadowbrook, 1984); and Sheila Kitzinger, *Giving Birth: How It Really Feels* (New York: The Noonday Press, Farrar, Straus and Giroux, 1989).

7. Tom Clark, "I Become a Father," *Progressive World* 22 (1969): 8–9.
8. Maurer and Maurer, *The World of the Newborn*, 53.
9. Ibid.
10. K. O'Driscoll, M. Foley, and D. MacDonald, "Active Management of Labor as an Alternative to Cesarean Section for Dystocia," *Obstetrics and Gynecology* 63 (1984): 485–90.
11. B. Jordan, *Birth in Four Cultures*, 23.
12. Marcha Flint, "Lockmi: An Indian Midwife," in *Anthropology of Human Birth*, ed. Margarita Artschwager Kay (Philadelphia: F. A. Davis Company, 1982), 213.
13. Marshall H. Klaus and John H. Kennell, *Parent-Infant Bonding*, 2nd ed. (New York: C. V. Mosby, 1982).
14. Aidan MacFarlane, *The Psychology of Childbirth* (Cambridge: Harvard University Press, 1977), 92.

5 The Expectant Father's Experience

1. There are now many delightful and competent books for expectant and new fathers on the market. See, for example, Ross D. Parke, *Fathers* (Cambridge: Harvard University Press, 1981); David Laskin, *Parents' Book for New Fathers* (New York: Ballantine Books, 1988); and our own book, *The Father: Mythology and Changing Roles* (Chicago: Chiron Press, 1988). For an excellent collection of professional articles, see Stanley H. Cath, Alan R. Gurwitt, and John Munder Ross, eds., *Father and Child: Developmental and Clinical Perspectives* (New York: Basil Blackwell, 1982).
2. W. H. Trehowan, "The Couvade Syndrome," *British Journal of Psychiatry* 111 (1965): 57–66.
3. See, for example, Henry Biller, "Father Absence and the Personality Development of the Male Child," *Developmental Psychology* 2 (1970): 181–201.

4. See Margaret Mead and Niles Newton, "Cultural Patterning of Perinatal Behavior," in *Childbearing: Its Social and Psychological Aspects*, ed. Steven A. Richardson and Alan F. Guttmacher (Baltimore: Williams & Wilkins, 1967), 142–244.

5. Engel, "An American Experience of Pregnancy and Childbirth in Japan," 83.

6. B. Jordan, *Birth in Four Cultures*, 24.

7. Ibid., 37.

8. Erik H. Erikson, *Childhood and Society* (New York: Norton, 1963), 55.

9. Ibid.

10. B. Jordan, *Birth in Four Cultures*, 38.

11. F. M. Dostoevsky, 1867 letter, in *The Notebooks for The Idiot*, ed. E. Wasiolek (Chicago: University of Chicago Press, 1967), 1.

12. Richard Rodgers and Oscar Hammerstein II, *Carousel*, in *Six Plays by Rodgers and Hammerstein* (New York: The Modern Library, 1959), 139–40.

13. Bob Dylan, "Father of Night," in *Writings and Drawings* (New York: Knopf, 1973), 296.

14. Bernstein and Kidd, "Childbearing in Japan," 102.

15. For a thorough study of the dreams of expectant fathers, see Alan Siegel, *Pregnant Dreams: Developmental Processes in the Manifest Dreams of Pregnant Fathers* (Ann Arbor: Dissertations International, 1982).

16. Quoted by columnist Herb Caen in the *San Francisco Chronicle*, 11 December 1989, B1.

17. Marsha Dawn Young, "An Exploration of Prenatal Paternal Bonding" (Ph.D. diss., The Fielding Institute, 1983).

18. George Bernard Shaw, *Man and Superman* (New York: Dodd, Mead, 1952), xix.

19. Bob Newhart, *Bob Newhart Faces Bob Newhart (Faces Bob Newhart)*, Warner Brothers Records #1517.

20. Bernstein and Kidd, "Childbearing in Japan," 102.

21. Greenberg, *The Birth of a Father* (New York: Avon Books, 1985), 12–13.

22. Ibid., 216.

6   *The Fourth Trimester*

1. For a very readable presentation of Winnicott's views of the early mother-infant relationship, see D. W. Winnicott, *Babies and Their Mothers*, ed. Clare Winnicott, Ray Shepherd, and Madeleine Davis (Reading, Massachusetts: Addison-Wesley Publishing Company, 1987).
2. Roberta Israeloff, *Coming to Terms* (New York: Penguin Books, 1984), 108.
3. M. W. O'Hara, "Social Support, Life Events, and Depression During Pregnancy and the Puerperium," *Archives of General Psychiatry* 43 (1986): 569. See also Luli Emmons Graetch, *A Study of Marital Variables as They Relate to Maternal Postpartum Mood* (Ph.D. diss., Pacific Graduate School of Psychology, 1988).
4. Soheir Morsy, "Childbirth in an Egyptian Village," in *Anthropology of Human Birth*, ed. Margarita Artschwager Kay (Philadelphia: F. A. Davis Company, 1982), 173.
5. Barbara Pillsbury, " 'Doing the Month': Confinement and Convalescence of Chinese Women After Childbirth," in *Anthropology of Human Birth*, ed. Margarita Artschwager Kay (Philadelphia: F. A. Davis Company, 1982).
6. Bernstein and Kidd, "Childbearing in Japan."
7. Pillsbury, " 'Doing the Month,' " 125.
8. Pediatric nurse practitioner Meg Zweibach, personal communication.
9. Pamela Jordan, "Laboring for Relevance: The Male Experience of Expectant and New Parenthood," *Nursing Research* 39 (1990): 15–16.
10. Reva Rubin, *Maternal Identity and the Maternal Experience* (New York: Springer Publishing Company, 1984), 109.

7   *Conclusion: Six Psychological Tasks
of the Childbearing Year*

1. Certain special conditions strongly affect the task of accepting a pregnancy. Most obviously, a couple that is adopting a baby has a special relationship to pregnancy. Commonly, they do

not know the biological mother of their child. Their preparation for parenthood occurs in the process of seeking the adoptive child. The recent trend toward pairing the biological mother with the adoptive parents more closely approximates the usual preparation for parenthood and gives the adoptive parents a chance to experience the pregnancy, at least vicariously. It also helps the biological mother integrate the pregnancy with her life experience and process her loss through an acknowledged mourning.

In another special case, a woman with a test-tube pregnancy may feel that the pregnancy is in the hands of the medical staff, and is less likely to incorporate the process fully into her psychology. Similarly, a woman who is afraid of an abnormality in her fetus or that she is at high risk for a miscarriage or who may still choose to have an abortion will not fully incorporate the pregnancy into her life.

2. P. Jordan, "Laboring for Relevance," 14.
3. O'Hara, "Social Support, Life Events, and Depression."
4. Rebecca S. Cohen and Sidney H. Weissman, "The Parenting Alliance," in *Parenthood: A Psychodynamic Perspective*, ed. Rebecca S. Cohen, Bertram J. Cohler, and Sidney H. Weissman (New York: The Guilford Press, 1984), 33–49.
5. Borg and Lasker, *When Pregnancy Fails*.
6. Israeloff, *Coming to Terms*, 118.
7. P. Jordan, "Laboring for Relevance," 17.

Bibliography

Badinter, Elisabeth. *Mother Love: Myth and Reality*. New York: Macmillan, 1981.

Bernstein, Gail Lee, and Yasue Aoki Kidd. "Childbearing in Japan." In *Anthropology of Human Birth*, edited by Margarita Artschwager Kay, 101–18. Philadelphia: F. A. Davis Company, 1982.

Bettelheim, Bruno. *A Good Enough Parent: A Book on Child-Rearing*. New York: Vintage Books, 1988.

Biller, Henry. "Father Absence and the Personality Development of the Male Child." *Developmental Psychology* 2 (1970): 181–201.

Bing, Elisabeth, and Libby Colman. *Having a Baby After Thirty*. New York: The Noonday Press, Farrar, Straus and Giroux, 1989.

——. *Making Love During Pregnancy*. New York: The Noonday Press, Farrar, Straus and Giroux, 1989.

Blatt, Robin J. R. *Prenatal Tests: What They Are, Their Benefits and Risks, and How to Decide Whether to Have Them or Not*. New York: Vintage Books, 1988.

Borg, Susan, and Judith Lasker. *When Pregnancy Fails.* New York: Bantam, 1988.

Boston Women's Health Collective. *Our Bodies, Ourselves.* New York: Simon and Schuster, 1971.

Bruch, Hilde. *Eating Disorders: Obesity, Anorexia Nervosa and the Person Within.* New York: Basic Books, 1973.

Caplan, Gerald. "Psychological Aspects of Maternity Care." *American Journal of Public Health* 47 (1954): 25–31.

Cath, Stanley H., Alan R. Gurwitt, and John Munder Ross, eds. *Father and Child: Developmental and Clinical Perspectives.* New York: Basil Blackwell, 1982.

Chodorow, Nancy. *The Reproduction of Mothering: Psychoanalysis and the Sociology of Gender.* Berkeley: University of California Press, 1978.

Clark, Tom. "I Become a Father." *Progressive World* 22 (1969): 1–12.

Cohen, Nancy Warner, and Lois J. Estner. *Silent Knife: Cesarean Prevention and Vaginal Birth After Cesarean.* Boston: Bergin & Garvey, Publishers, 1983.

Cohen, Rebecca S., and Sidney H. Weissman. "The Parenting Alliance." In *Parenthood: A Psychodynamic Perspective,* edited by Rebecca S. Cohen, Bertram J. Cohler, and Sidney H. Weissman, 33–49. New York: The Guilford Press, 1988.

Colman, Arthur D. "Psychological State during First Pregnancy." *American Journal of Orthopsychiatry* 39 (1960): 788–97.

———. "Psychology of a First Baby Group." *International Journal of Group Psychotherapy* 21 (1971): 74–83.

Colman, Arthur D., and Libby Lee Colman. *The Father: Mythology and Changing Roles.* Chicago: Chiron Press, 1988.

———. *Pregnancy: The Psychological Experience.* New York: The Seabury Press, 1971.

Cowan, C. P., P. Cowan, G. Henning, E. Garrett, W. S. Coysh, H. Curtis-Bowles, and A. J. Bowles. "Transitions to Parenthood: His, Hers, and Theirs." *The Journal of Family Issues* 6 (1985): 451–81.

DelliQuadri, Lyn, and Kati Breckenridge. *The New Mother Care: Helping Yourself Through the Emotional and Physical Transitions of Motherhood.* Los Angeles: Jeremy Tarcher, 1977.

Dick-Read, Grantly. *Childbirth without Fear.* Revised and edited by Helen Wessel and Harlan Ellis. New York: Harper & Row, 1985.

Eliot, Alexander, with contributions by Mircea Eliade and Joseph Campbell. *Myths.* New York: McGraw-Hill Book Company, 1976.

Engel, Nancy Sharts. "An American Experience of Pregnancy and Childbirth in Japan." *Birth* 16 (1989): 81–86.

Erikson, Erik H. *Childhood and Society.* New York: Norton, 1963.

Flint, Marcha. "Lockmi: An Indian Midwife." In *Anthropology of Human Birth*, edited by Margarita Artschwager Kay, 211–20. Philadelphia: F. A. Davis Company, 1982.

Friedland, Ronnie, and Carol Kort. *The Mothers' Book: Shared Experiences.* Boston: Houghton Mifflin Company, 1981.

Gabrielson, I. W., L. V. Klerman, J. B. Currie, N. C. Tyler, and J. F. Jakel. "Attempted Suicide Among Pregnant Teenagers." *American Journal of Public Health* 60 (1968): 2289–2301.

Genevie, Louis, and Eva Margolies. *The Motherhood Report: How Women Feel about Being Mothers.* New York: McGraw-Hill Book Company, 1989.

Gillman, R. D. "The Dreams of Pregnant Women and Maternal Adaptation." *American Journal of Orthopsychiatry* 38 (1968): 688–92.

Graetch, Luli Emmons. "A Study of Marital Variables as They Relate to Maternal Postpartum Mood." Ph.D. diss., Pacific Graduate School of Psychology, 1988.

Greenberg, Martin. *The Birth of a Father.* New York: Avon Books, 1985.

Hall, Elizabeth. "When Does Life Begin: A Conversation with Clifford Grobstein." *Psychology Today*, September 1989, 42–46.

Hanson, Shirley M. H., and Frederick W. Bozett. *Dimensions of Fatherhood*. Beverly Hills: Sage Publications, 1985.

Hees-Stauthamer, Jellemieke C. *The First Pregnancy: An Integrating Principle in Female Psychology*. Ann Arbor: UMI Research Press, 1985.

Israeloff, Roberta. *Coming to Terms*. New York: Penguin Books, 1984.

Jordan, Brigitte. *Birth in Four Cultures: A Crosscultural Investigation of Childbirth in Yucatan, Holland, Sweden and the United States*. Montreal: Eden Press Women's Publications, 1978.

Jordan, Pamela. "Laboring for Relevance: The Male Experience of Expectant and New Parenthood." *Nursing Research* 39 (1990): 11–16.

Kitzinger, Sheila. *Giving Birth: How It Really Feels*. New York: The Noonday Press, Farrar, Straus and Giroux, 1989.
———. *Women as Mothers: How They See Themselves in Different Cultures*. New York: Random House, 1978.

Klaus, Marshall H., and John H. Kennell. *Parent-Infant Bonding*. 2nd ed. New York: C. V. Mosby, 1982.

Lamb, Michael E., ed. *The Role of the Father in Child Development*. New York: John Wiley & Sons, 1976.

Lang, Andrew, ed. "Rapunzel." In *The Red Fairy Book*, 282–85. New York: Dover Publications, 1966.

Lasch, Christopher. *The Culture of Narcissism: American Life in an Age of Diminishing Expectations*. New York: Warner Books, 1979.

Laskin, David. *Parents' Book for New Fathers*. New York: Ballantine Books, 1988.

Leifer, Myra. *Psychological Effects of Motherhood: A Study of First Pregnancy*. New York: Praeger, 1980.

Lynn, David B. *The Father: His Role in Child Development*. Monterey, California: Brooks/Cole Publishing Company, 1974.

MacFarlane, Aidan. *The Psychology of Childbirth.* Cambridge: Harvard University Press, 1977.

Margolis, Maxine. *Mothers and Such: Views of American Women and Why They Changed.* Berkeley: University of California Press, 1984.

Mariesking, Helen I. "Cesarean Section in the United States: Has It Changed Since 1979?" *Birth* 16 (December 1989): 196– 202.

Masters, William H., and Virginia E. Johnson. *Human Sexual Response.* Boston: Little, Brown and Company, 1966.

Maurer, Daphne, and Charles Maurer. *The World of the Newborn.* New York: Basic Books, 1988.

May, Katherine Antle. "Three Phases in the Development of Father Involvement in Pregnancy." *Nursing Research* 31 (1982): 337–42.

Mead, Margaret, and Niles Newton. "Cultural Patterning of Perinatal Behavior." In *Childbearing: Its Social and Psychological Aspects,* edited by Steve A. Richardson and Alan F. Guttmacher, 142–244. Baltimore: Williams & Wilkins, 1967.

Menning, Barbara Eck. *Infertility.* Englewood Cliffs, New Jersey: Prentice-Hall, 1977.

Mercer, Ramona T. *First-Time Motherhood: Experiences from Teens to Forties.* New York: Springer Publishing Company, 1986.

Mintz, Steven, and Susan Kellogg. *Domestic Revolutions: A Social History of American Family Life.* New York: The Free Press, Macmillan, 1988.

Morsy, Soheir. "Childbirth in an Egyptian Village." In *Anthropology of Human Birth,* edited by Margarita Artschwager Kay, 147–74. Philadelphia: F. A. Davis Company, 1982.

Nathanson, Sue. *Soul Crisis.* New York: New American Library, 1989.

O'Driscoll, K., M. Foley, and D. MacDonald. "Active Management of Labor as an Alternative to Cesarean Section for Dystocia." *Obstetrics and Gynecology* 63 (1984): 485–90.

O'Hara, M. W. "Social Support, Life Events, and Depression During Pregnancy and the Puerperium." *Archives of General Psychiatry* 43 (1986): 569–73.

Parke, Ross D. *Fathers.* Cambridge: Harvard University Press, 1981.

Parks, J. "Emotional Reactions to Pregnancy." *American Journal of Obstetrics and Gynecology* 62 (1951): 339.

Peterson, Gayle, and Lewis Mehl. *Pregnancy as Healing.* Berkeley: Mindbody Press, 1984.

Pillsbury, Barbara. " 'Doing the Month': Confinement and Convalescence of Chinese Women After Childbirth." In *Anthropology of Human Birth*, edited by Margarita Artschwager Kay, 119–46. Philadelphia: F. A. Davis Company, 1982.

Pruett, Kyle D. *The Nurturing Father: Journey Toward the Complete Man.* New York: Warner Books, 1987.

Rabuzzi, Kathryn Allen. *Motherself: A Mythic Analysis of Motherhood.* Bloomington: Indiana University Press, 1988.

Radcliffe, Walter. *Milestones in Midwifery.* Bristol, England: Wright, 1967.

Rosen, Mortimer, and Lillian Thomas. *The Cesarean Myth: Choosing the Best Way to Have Your Baby.* New York: Penguin, 1989.

Rosenberg, A. J., and E. Silver. "The Psychiatrist and Therapeutic Abortion." *California Medicine* 102 (1965): 407–11.

Rothman, Barbara Katz. *The Tentative Pregnancy: Prenatal Diagnosis and the Future of Motherhood.* New York: Viking, 1986.

Rubin, Reva. *Maternal Identity and the Maternal Experience.* New York: Springer Publishing Company, 1984.

Saltzman, S., and T. Schneidman. "Psychological Study of the Woman." *A Demonstration Project in Prenatal and Early Postnatal Adaptation, Final Report.* Washington, D.C.: U.S. Department of Health, 1968.

Sandler, Merton, ed. *Mental Illness in Pregnancy and the Puerperium.* Oxford: Oxford University Press, 1978.

Scott, Lucy, and Meredith Joan Angwin. *Time Out for Motherhood: A Guide for Today's Working Woman to the Financial, Emotional and Career Aspects of Having a Baby*. Los Angeles: Jeremy Tarcher, 1986.

Shereshefsky, Pauline, and Leon J. Yarrow. *Psychological Aspects of a First Pregnancy and Early Postnatal Adaptation*. New York: Raven Press, 1973.

Siegel, Alan. *Pregnant Dreams: Developmental Processes in the Manifest Dreams of Pregnant Fathers*. Ann Arbor: Dissertations International, 1982.

Simkin, Penny, Janet Whalley, and Ann Keppler. *Pregnancy, Childbirth and the Newborn: A Complete Guide for Expectant Parents*. New York: Meadowbrook, 1984.

Stukane, Eileen. *The Dream Worlds of Pregnancy*. New York: Quill, 1985.

Sullivan, Bonnie. *The Cesarean Childbirth Experience: A Practical and Reassuring Guide for Partners and Professionals*. Boston: Beacon Press, 1986.

Tobin, Sidney M. "Emotional Depression during Pregnancy." *Obstetrics and Gynecology* 10 (1957): 677–81.

Trehowan, W. H. "The Couvade Syndrome." *British Journal of Psychiatry* 111 (1965): 57–66.

Verny, Thomas, M.D., and John Kelly. *The Secret Life of the Unborn Child*. New York: Summit Books, 1981.

Wessel, Helen. *Natural Childbirth and the Christian Family*. New York: Harper & Row, 1963.

Winnicott, D. W. *Babies and Their Mothers*. Edited by Clare Winnicott, Ray Shepherd, and Madeleine Davis. Reading, Massachusetts: Addison-Wesley Publishing Company, 1987.

Wolkind, S., and E. Zajicek, eds. *Pregnancy: A Psychological and Social Study*. New York: Grune & Stratton, 1981.

Young, Marsha Dawn. "An Exploration of Prenatal Paternal Bonding." Ph.D. diss., The Fielding Institute, 1983.

Index